T5-CQC-556

CLARA M. CHANEY

Parent Training,
Glen Haven Achievement Center,
Ft. Collins, Colorado

NEWELL C. KEPHART

Director,
Glen Haven Achievement Center,
Ft. Collins, Colorado

MOTORIC AIDS TO PERCEPTUAL TRAINING

CHARLES E. MERRILL PUBLISHING COMPANY

Columbus, Ohio   *A Bell & Howell Company*

THE SLOW LEARNER SERIES

edited by Newell C. Kephart, Ph.D.

© 1968 by Charles E. Merrill Publishing Company, Columbus, Ohio. All rights reserved. No part of this book may be reproduced in any form, by mimeograph or any other means, without permission in writing from the publisher.

Library of Congress Catalog Card Number: 68-8630

ISBN 0-675-09594-8

6 7 8 9 10–74

Printed in the United States of America

Preface

Initial training activities with children who display learning disabilities frequently involve motor learnings and the development of more adequate motor responses. Such activities, however, are not designed to teach pure motor skills. Rather they must take into account the more complex perceptual-motor responses which are occurring concomitantly in the child and must be directed toward the enhancement of these more complex functions. At the same time, inadequate motor responses may be obstructing perceptual learning, and perceptual training may be difficult or impossible in the face of such motor inadequacy.

It is in this sense that the concept of motor concomitants of perceptual training should be interpreted. An attempt is made to aid the child in the learning of those generalized motor responses which contribute to his development of skills in the perceptual and conceptual areas. The aspects of motor activities for concern as well as the activities themselves are selected for their contribution to this overall development. In like manner, learning activities prescribed are selected with this purpose in mind.

It is the initial aspects of such a sequential development to which *Motoric Aids to Perceptual Training* is directed. The total range of learning interferences in the child and the total attack upon these problems should be kept in mind as the book is read.

CLARA M. CHANEY

NEWELL C. KEPHART

Acknowledgments

The material contained in *Motoric Aids to Perceptual Training* was originally presented at a workshop sponsored by the Division of Special Education of the Wisconsin State Department of Public Instruction. The proceedings of this conference were subsequently published as Bulletin 4A of the Division of Special Education, Madison, Wisconsin, 1963. The authors wish to express their gratitude to this division for permission to republish that material.

The original presentation has been revised and augmented in the present volume through the addition of material developed at the Achievement Center for Children, Purdue University, during the intervening years. Much credit is due the staff of the Achievement Center for their contributions to the development of this new material.

The authors also wish to thank Stephen F. Miles for the photographs herein.

C. M. C.

N. C. K.

Contents

section 1

chapter 1

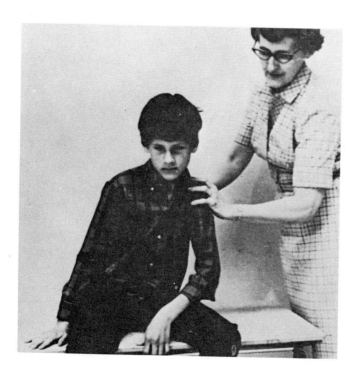

Adjustive movements maintain balance against resistance.

Motor-Perceptual Learning

For many years, workers in the field of child development have identified stages in the growth and development of children. It is customary to talk of sequences of development in many areas of the child's activity, and elaborate normative studies have revealed the age at which specific activities can normally be expected to appear (3). For the most part these studies have been concerned with specific performances or with specific skills. When the performances investigated have become complex, their complexity was frequently the result of the combination of a large number of specific skills.

It would seem possible to view development in the child, not so much as a sequence of specific skills and performances, but as the sequential development of certain basic generalizations. Such a view of development shifts our attention from the specific performances of the child toward the observation of general characteristics of behavior; from skills in specific tasks to more generalized behaviors contributing to performance in many tasks. Such a shift in point of view seems to be of particular significance in considerations of the brain injured child since, as has been repeatedly pointed out, the effect of a brain injury in early childhood is not so much to interfere with specific performances as to make difficult the development of such generalized responses as form perception and concept formation. Let us consider the development of such generalizations in what is probably the most basic of all the areas of development in the child.

MOTOR SYSTEM

Embryologically, the first neurological system to develop is the motor system (1, 6, 12). The motor system is laid down and becomes functional before the perceptual system is ready. The association system is the last to develop and is built upon the two previous systems which are already operating.

The first learnings of the human organism are motor learnings. In early childhood, mental and physical activities are closely related as Jersild (8) points out, and motor activities play a major role in intellectual development.

Thus, both embryologically and psychologically, the motor system is there first. It represents the initial system in the developmental hierarchy. As with all other developments in nature, more advanced systems do not begin from scratch but represent expansions and elaborations of existing systems. In the human organism, the system which, because of its prior development, must be used as the basis for such expansion and elaboration is the motor system. It is logical, therefore, to expect that the earliest generalizations with which we must be concerned in child training are motor generalizations.

MOTOR LEARNING

Physical growth and motor development proceed according to two general principles (10). The first of these is progression from general to specific action, from gross to specific refined control. The second is in some respects its opposite: development from specific refined control to general systems of movement. The undifferentiated general wave of movement of the former principle must be differentiated into an integrated series of patterned movements of parts. The highly individualized and specific reflexes of the second principle must be integrated and organized into elaborated reflex systems (11). In both cases, development and learning must supply organization and system: in the former by differentiation, in the latter by summation. Generalized motor behaviors supplant amorphic movements on the one hand and isolated reflex responses on the other.

Out of the generalized undifferentiated movement, more specific responses arise under the influence of development and learning. Whereas initially the arm moved only in complete subjugation to the trunk, for example, now it is able to move independently of the trunk. Specific parts and specific muscle groups can be used for their own purposes without the involvement of the entire organism in the movement.

There are two general principles governing such differentiation of specific responses. The first of these is the cephalo-caudal principle which refers to the fact that growth and motor development proceed, in general, from the head end to the tail end of the organism. Thus, the first effective motor control is exerted over the muscles which lift the head, and the first part which can be moved independently is the head. Later, similar differentiation takes place in the arm, shoulder, and abdominal musculature. Finally, differentiation of movements of the legs, ankles, and feet occurs. Independent control of the parts and specific movements of the parts develop in a head to tail direction.

The second principle of differentiation is the proximo-distal, which refers to the fact that growth and motor development proceed from the axis of the body outward to the periphery. Thus the infant's early reaching responses are accomplished by gross movements from the shoulder with the arm and hand used as a unit. Independent use of wrist or finger movements does not occur until well along in his first year.

According to these two principles, then, development and learning result in the differentiation of specific responses out of the early undifferentiated mass movement. It is, of course, important that such differentiation occur; only through such a process do independent control and independent movement of parts become possible. However, it is also important that differentiation takes place according to pattern and follows the two principles outlined above. It is through differentiation *in pattern* that the developing specific movements and skills are maintained as a part of a total organism and exist as an overall repertory of motor responses rather than a mere collection of independent skills. It is through differentiation *in pattern* that the child builds up a structured motor response system.

It is in the development of such a *structured* system that the brain injured child frequently encounters difficulty. The development of a structure or pattern is a complex process, depending as it does on both a quantity of responses, and more importantly, upon an organization of these responses. Responses must not only exist but interconnections between them must be preserved. It seems obvious that such structuring requires the simultaneous functioning of much larger areas of the cortex than does the simple performance of an isolated movement. Therefore, the interference resulting from an interruption of activities of the central nervous system would be expected to be more marked in such diffuse functions than in more isolated functions. The probability of interference is increased as the function begins to involve more diffuse areas of the cortex.

SPLINTERING

One can imagine the child with learning disorders beginning the process of differentiation in a normal manner. At some point in the process, the interference from the involvement becomes apparent and the next step in the differentiation process becomes difficult. He therefore falls behind in his learning and differentiation stops (either temporarily or more permanently). The pressures for learning bearing upon the child from outside, however, do not stop. These outside pressures continue without regard to the fact that the child has encountered a difficulty. The pressures increase in severity and in level just as though the child's development had continued at the normal pace. His blocked learning is not recognized, nor is any account taken of the fact that he has not been able to advance through the differentiation process. At some point the external stresses become so strong that a temporizing adaptation is necessary. The child, therefore, suspends the pattern of differentiation, gives increased attention to the part or parts under stress, and learns to manipulate this part in the manner required by the outside pressure. In so doing, however, he learns an isolated skill not related to the more generalized learning which has taken place earlier. He develops *a splinter skill* which permits him to satisfy the outside agent but has little or no connection with anything else which is going on in the organism.

An example may make more clear what can happen. A ten-year-old boy was asked to write his name on the chalkboard. He placed his wrist on the board, and using only the fingers (as though he were writing with pencil and paper), began the process of writing his name. It was noticed that each stroke of each letter was made independently. Thus, he made the first stroke of the first letter, stopped, made the second stroke, stopped, and so on throughout the performance. When it was completed he turned and said to the examiner "I can write my name. I have memorized the movements."

It seems possible that this child experienced a difficulty in the differentiation process somewhere before the precise movements of the fingers had been differentiated out of the mass. However, the home or the school or someone had insisted that he learn to write. When this pressure became sufficiently great, he suspended general development, and to accomplish a specific task, learned to use his fingers to form certain letters. The only way he could perform the task was to memorize a prescribed series of movements. In the process, these fine movements of the fingers were splintered off from any other activities of the organism with the result that he could accomplish them under one condition and one condition only. Thus, if not allowed to rest his wrist on the board as he had done on the paper, he could not write his name. In like manner, these finger movements were not related to other parts of the body, such as wrist and arm, or to the movements of these other body parts. It was necessary, with this boy, to go back to the point where differentiation had departed from pattern, restore the sequence, and help him to develop a structure of movements. Only then could he learn to write in a more normal fashion.

When differentiation of specific movements out of the initial global mass proceeds normally, the concept of the whole is retained. The specific movement retains an aspect of belonging to the whole. In this way a structure is developed in which interrelationships are preserved so that a patterned whole results.

It seems probable that such splintering occurs frequently in the learning of the child with neurological impairment. Our teaching methods and our curriculum materials assume that development has occurred *in pattern*. These educational techniques, therefore, also assume that the child's behavior is based on the fundamental generalizations normally resulting from such development. In the case of the brain injured child, these fundamental assumptions may not be met. Continued reapplication of methods designed for normal children or continued drill on specific tasks considered important either for their own sakes or as "tool" skills may force the child to substitute a specific skill for a more generalized one. Although such drill may result in immediate performance, the long range problems of the child may be increased instead of decreased.

It may well prove more economical, both in terms of the teaching program and in terms of the child's development, to divert attention temporarily from the specific performance to the methods by which the child is accomplishing the task. It may be necessary to spend initial effort on the development of the fundamental generalization in order to conserve time later when many specific tasks must be taught.

At the same time that differentiation of specific movements out of the mass is going on, a second system of movements is developing. Initial reflex responses are being integrated into more complex functions.

As a result of development and learning, simple reflexes become elaborated. Additional elements of movement are added to the initial response, and reflex responses are becoming related to each other. The initial response is expanded to include a larger series of movements. At the same time the stimuli which can elicit the reflex are being expanded. Instead of a specific stimulus, a cluster of stimuli may be used to set off the response. The end result of such development is the formation of a pattern among reflex responses. If these patterns are extensive enough, a structure of reflexes results which is similar to the structure resulting from differentiation out of the mass.

Two highly structured repositories of movement responses are, therefore, developed: one resulting from patterned differentiation of specific movements out of a generalized mass; the other resulting from a patterned integration of specific responses into structured wholes. These two structures combine into a total organized movement repertory.

MOTOR GENERALIZATION

The individual movements resulting from the combination of structures become combined into movement patterns. Such patterns are series of individual movements which produce an overt behavior. Thus walking is a series of specific movements performed in succession and synchronized with each other in time (4). The result is an overt behavior which moves the body through space in a prescribed manner. When this walking pattern has been achieved, it becomes automatic, and as long as there is no interference with the specific movements, it can be performed without undue attention to the processes.

Frequently, however, there is an outside interference with the specific movements in the pattern. Thus, in the walking pattern, the child may encounter an obstacle in his path which makes it impossible to put one foot in front of the other in the customary manner. If the walking pattern is the only motor response available to him, he must give direct attention to the movements which he will make and the manner in which he will make them in order to surmount the obstacle. Motor patterns, then, being relatively inflexible, do not permit continuous alteration for the purpose of adjusting to the outside demands of the task.

When a number of such patterns have been developed, the child organizes them around certain purposes or functions. Thus a series of movement patterns concerned with movement of the body through space will become clustered together to form a locomotor generalization. All or most of the movements concerned with this function will cluster together and become related one to another. Within this cluster, the child can move from one pattern to another freely and without undue attention to the changes in overt movement which are required.

The movement generalization thus becomes a repertory of movement patterns available for a given type of purpose. Since the patterns are related through the generalization, the same type of interchangeability and integration exists among them as exists among the isolated movements within the movement pattern. The child can shift readily between patterns to meet the demands of the situation. Thus attention is freed from the movement itself and made available for the purpose of the movement. A child with a locomotor generalization has no difficulty surmounting the obstacle mentioned above which proved a difficulty for the child with only the walking pattern. He can now merely shift from walking to jumping, hopping, or whatever may be necessary. Since the generalization takes care of the necessary movements, the child's attention can be directed solely to the purpose of the movement. Thus attention is not interrupted by the obstacle but can be maintained throughout. There are four such motor generalizations which are felt to be of particular significance in education (2). The first of these is *balance and posture*.

BALANCE AND POSTURE

Every object in the child's universe is related to every other object in space. These relationships, however, are not absolute; they are relative. They are dependent upon the position of the observer and the direction of the observation. The letters in a word, for example, run from left to right, if you look down on the page in the customary position. If, however, you hold the page up to the light and look through it from behind, the letters run from right to left. The spatial relationships of the letters are dependent upon the position of the observer. What is true of such formalized relationships is also true of all relationships between objects in space. Among all this mass of interrelationships, there is, for the human organism on the planet earth, one constant. That constant is the force of gravity. Gravity exerts a constant force in a constant direction. It, therefore, becomes the zero point or the point of origin for any systematic set of spatial relationships. Adults use the three dimensions of Euclidean space as the system by which they organize these relationships. The point of intersection of the three coordinates of Euclidean space and, hence, the point of origin for the system is the line of gravity through the observer's body.

Before any spatial system can be developed, this zero point must be established. Through the activities of balance and posture, the child determines where the line of gravity is and the direction of its force. Only when this knowledge is firmly established can he proceed to the development of coordinates of the space around him. Not only is it necessary that the child identify the line of gravity but, if his spatial system is to be stable, he must know at all times where he is in relation to gravity. He must, therefore, learn to identify the line of gravity through his own body and become constantly aware of the relationship between the position of his body in space and the direction of this force. Many children, who do not have such a firm relationship to gravity, gain the impression when they change position (such as going from standing to lying) that it was not their body which changed position but rather that space rotated around them. A firm generalization relative to gravity, through balance and posture, is required for the development of a spatial structure in the child. This generalization must be sufficiently flexible to permit the child to move, but at the same time it must be sufficiently firm so that he maintains at all times an awareness of gravity and its effect.

LOCOMOTION

The second motor generalization is that of *locomotion.* Locomotion includes those activities which result in moving the body through space, such as walking, running, hopping, jumping, rolling, etc. It is with these activities that the child investigates the relationships *between* objects in space. Through such investigations he will build up a systematic space structure within which all objects within his awareness at any given moment are included and the relationships between them maintained. Spatial directions and spatial orientation can be expected to develop through such exploration. Initially, these will be egocentrically oriented. The child will be able to relate any object to his own position. Later, they will become more objective so that he can relate the position of any object to that of any other object. Still later, they will become fully structured so that all objects occupy a position on a spatial matrix with the three Euclidean coordinates as its principle axes. In this last stage, the organization of words on a page of print or of problems on a page of arithmetic will become meaningful.

In order to establish such a space structure, consistent information about the relationships involved is required. It is difficult to establish a structure if the data are presented in a haphazard or random fashion. The bases of the structure are much more clear if the data follow some pattern. It is through a locomotor generalization that the child maintains consistency in the gathering of such spatial information. When the attention can be directed solely toward the information and when the pattern of the exploration can be determined ahead of time, intentionally consistent information can be obtained. When, however, the exploration is interrupted from time to time by the need to attend to the mechanics of movement or when exploration must be limited to those areas where no obstacles which might disrupt movement are present, a consistent body of information is difficult to obtain. A thorough space structure is a very extensive system of information. Both quantitatively and qualitatively its development requires certain consistent series of information. The locomotor generalization is, therefore, very significant to education because of its effect upon the early information gathering functions.

CONTACT

The third generalization is that of *contact*. It is with the contact skills that the child investigates the relationships within objects. They are the skills of manipulation by which the child handles objects and explores their nature. In the human organism, contact skills primarily involve the hand since this is the most efficient part for manipulation.

There are three aspects to the contact activities: *reach*, by which contact is made with an object; *grasp*, by which contact is maintained while the manipulatory activities are completed; and *release*, by which this contact is broken and the child is free to proceed to another exploration. The skill involved in each of these aspects is to some degree independent of that in the other aspects. Thus the early attempts at contact displayed by the young infant result in the hand contacting an object but do not yet permit that contact to be maintained. The grasp function requires skills somewhat different from those of the reach function, and these latter abilities have not yet been developed. For the purposes of manipulation, it is necessary that all the aspects of contact be present and that they be related to one another. If grasp is not synchronized with reach, it may occur too soon or too late. In either event, the objective of manipulation is lost. It is through a very fine synchronous interplay between these aspects that continuous, uninterrupted exploration of objects through manipulation is possible. Such an interplay results when the skills involved combine into a motor generalization which permits their guidance by the purpose of the activity.

The importance of manipulative activities to learning has been repeatedly stressed by workers in the fields of child development and early childhood education (7). These manipulatory explorations lay the foundation for the more advanced skills of form perception and figure ground relationships so important in classroom activities. The child observes through manipulation the relationships between the parts of an object, which will become the elements of a figure, and between the object and its surround, contrasting the figure with the ground.

As with locomotion, it is important that these manipulatory explorations be consistent and uninterrupted. Through consistent exploration a consistent body of information concerning the object is generated. Through continuous exploration a complete body of information is generated. Both of these factors aid greatly in the development of a systematic body of information concerning the object and its surround. For future learning, it is the information which is important. Therefore, the motor activities involved must be sufficiently developed and adequately organized so that attention can be almost exclusively directed toward the information which is being supplied.

RECEIPT AND PROPULSION

Through balance and posture the child developed a point of origin for the relationships in the environment around him. Through locomotion he explored the relationships between objects in that environment. With contact he explored the relationships within objects. He can, therefore, deal with a static universe. However, many of the relationships with which he is required to deal within his environment involve movement. An object moves in relationship to other objects. He requires a method of investigating movement within his environment and the changing relationships produced by such movement. This final set of relationships he explores through the generalization of receit and propulsion.

The skills of receipt include those activities with which he relates to an object moving toward him, by interposing his body or a part of his body in the path of the movement. Such activities as catching, trapping, stopping, and the like are involved. Propulsion involves those activities with which he relates to an object moving away from him. Such activities as pushing, throwing, batting, and the like are involved. Through an integration of these two sets of information, he learns to relate to objects moving laterally to himself or in planes other than those his body occupies.

The relativity of movement is revealed by such exploration. When an object moves, movement is attributed to the object which is considered to move in front of a ground. Without such appreciation, it is impossible to determine whether the object is moving in front of the ground or the ground is moving out from behind the object.

You have had the experience of sitting in a railroad train when a train on the next track starts to move. It is difficult to determine whether your train is moving in one direction or the other train is moving in the opposite direction. It is the same with a moving object and a ground. Many children behave as though they thought that the ground was moving away from behind the object. Such relativities can be sorted out and the movement attributed to the correct source through consistent exploration of moving objects. Such exploration is possible through the motor activities of the receipt and propulsion generalization.

Because of the relativity involved, an adequate body of information concerning movement must be very extensive. The long period through which children are enchanted by ball play and similar activities indicates the extent of the problem and the time required to solve it. Consistency and continuity of information are particularly important since the variables which must be investigated and interrelated are numerous. The perceptual changes related to changes in distance of an object illustrate the complications involved in the development of generalizations concerning movement (9). When these changes incorporate systematic variation due to movement, the problem is further complicated.

EXPLORATION

One of the primary learning tasks of the young child is that of obtaining and storing information concerning the environment around him. In the early stages of such learning it is the physical nature of the environment and the physical relationships within it which concern him. Such information is gathered through exploration: exploration with the hand for relationships within objects; exploration through locomotion for relationships between objects. Such exploration requires movement, and it is the movement which determines what information and what successions of information will be obtained. Movement, therefore, becomes essential to the gathering of information concerning the environment.

If information so gathered is to become useful in the solution of problems, it must be organized and integrated so that in any problem situation those data pertinent to the problem will be available and those not pertinent will not intrude on the problem solving process. For such an organization of information, systematized storage is required. Information must be stored in terms of certain classifications and in terms of certain principles which pertain to the relationships in the environment itself. Systematic storage is greatly aided by systematic gathering of initial information. Thus systematic exploration greatly aids subsequent development of organized bodies of information about the environment.

Systematic exploration, however, requires uninterrupted exploratory activities. Throughout the exploration, the child's attention must be given to the information which is being generated. If his attention must be diverted to the question of how the exploration will be made, the continuity of the information is interrupted and its systematic nature is less obvious. Consider the child who explores the space across a room and the spatial relationships of the objects occupying that space. If he starts to locomote across the room but encounters an obstacle, and if he has only motor patterns with which to move, he must divert his attention from the relationships which he is observing and, for a greater or lesser period of time, direct it to the problem of moving in the face of the obstacle. When the exploration is completed, there will be a gap in the information. The relationships between the objects being observed will be continuous for a part of the time and then will become discontinuous while attention had to be shifted to the problem of movement. The total exploration is incomplete, and it is the systematic nature of the information which is most affected as a result. Such a child may well have difficulty building up a systematic body of spatial information and, because of this difficulty, have trouble developing a space structure within which to organize the spatial relations around him.

For systematic exploration, motor generalizations are necessary. Motor patterns are not sufficiently flexible to permit continuity of exploration. With motor patterns only, the child must from time to time interrupt the exploration in order to continue the movement. The purpose of the movement is thus disrupted and, where basic information about the environment is concerned, the systematic nature of that information is obscured. Motor generalization is therefore very important to education since it is with these functions that the basic structure of information is laid. Future, more complex information systems will be built upon this basic structure and will, in turn, take their structure from it. Defects in the basic structure can be expected to be reflected later in the more complex structures.

BODY IMAGE

Early information about the environment comes through contacts between the child and the outside world. This interaction can be directed and determined only if the child himself moves and thus initiates the contact. Without movement, such contacts as may occur are largely random and are externally determined. When the child moves, he is able, at least in part, to determine what the nature of the contact will be and thus what information it will deliver. It is then possible to produce consistency in the incoming information and to check and re-check until a systematic body of information is achieved.

For such purposes, movement is necessary. At all times, however, the movement itself is subordinate to the information generated through the movement. The human organism is highly flexible and has many methods available for obtaining a given piece of information. It follows, therefore, that no one specific movement or movement pattern is essential to the development of information. If one movement is difficult or impossible, there may exist another movement which will generate the same information. The emphasis is therefore upon systems of movement which make available to the child many ways of verifying or generating information. Specific skills are of secondary importance. The child requires a large repertory of movement possibilities, none of which is performed with an exceptional degree of skill, but all of which are performed sufficiently well to provide information. These specific movements must likewise be organized into clusters or groupings which serve particular purposes, and the purpose outweighs the performance.

Although specific skills are not the primary consideration in the motor development of the child, at least as it relates to the problems of education, it is important that the child know what he can do and what types of vironmental contact can emanate from this point of origin while its movements and possibilities for contact is included in his body image.

As used here, body image refers to the child's awareness of his body and its capabilities. It includes the answer to four major questions: What are the parts? What can they do? How do you make them do it? What space do they occupy while doing it?

The point of origin for all the relationships within the environment lies within the body at the line of gravity, as has been pointed out. In any systematic exploration, it is necessary to know what the point of origin is and what is happening to it. The child needs to know what types of environmental contact can emanate from this point of origin while its locus is still maintained. He needs to know the nature of the continuing relationships between the point of origin and the environmental contacts. Therefore, it is important for him to know what his body can do and how it is organized during the performance. Since the point of origin is related to the problem of space, it is important to know what spatial changes occur during a contact. To maintain the point of origin intact and to develop a system which is consistent around this point, the child needs a strong body image which can inform him at all times of the nature of himself within the environment.

LATERALITY

A second important consideration growing out of the child's motor explorations is that of laterality. Laterality is an appreciation within the body of the difference between right and left. It is this directional differentiation which forms the basis for the lateral dimension of space. Just as an appreciation of the direction of the force of gravity lays the basis for the vertical direction, so laterality lays the basis for the horizontal direction.

The human nervous system is roughly divided into two halves: a right half and a left half. Impulses controlling activities on the right side of the body originate in the left hemisphere of the brain, cross over to the right side, and are conveyed to muscles. In like manner, tactual and kinesthetic sensations resulting from movements on the right side are conveyed up the spinal cord where they cross over to the left side of the cortex. There are many interconnections and many intercommunication channels between the two systems so that the cleavage is not as sharp as indicated here. However, in general there is one subsystem for the right half of the body and another subsystem for the left. This arrangement makes of the organism an excellent right-left detection device. Information is supplied regarding the side of the body engaged in any activity and also regarding happenings on each side of the body.

The mere anatomical existence of such a system, however, does not imply its operation. The child must learn how to use the system. He must learn to interpret the information delivered by it. By analyzing many movements and their results he must learn which side is moving and when it is moving. In like manner, he must learn to interpret tactual and kinesthetic impulses from the two sides in terms of the location of the stimulus.

From such comparisons the child develops a sort of right-left gradient which tells him which side of his body is active and how far from the midline the activity lies. Out of this gradient will grow the horizontal dimension of space. This dimension will at first exist within the child's body, incorporated into the body of motor information which he has built up. Later it will be projected, through perceptual activities, onto outside spaces and objects so that they too have a right and left dimension. The development of laterality requires a great many experiences from which the two sides can be compared: bilateral experiences, unilateral experiences, alternating experiences. Careful attention to the differences between such experiences can result in the development of a system of information which imparts to any event a right-left quality.

PERCEPTUAL-MOTOR MATCH

While the child is actively exploring his environment, he is also receiving perceptual information. The external sense organs are responding to patterns of energy from the environment and are conveying these patterns to the central nervous system. When a pattern of energy strikes a sense organ, neural impulses are generated. By virtue of the anatomical nature of the organ, these neural patterns are related to the outside pattern of energy. They thus reflect what exists in the environment. However, at this early stage of development, they are not related to anything which is going on inside the organism. They are meaningless in so far as the child's activities are concerned. It is necessary to relate these meaningless patterns to more meaningful activities within the organism so that they can be translated and become useful in determining responses.

A correlation between incoming perceptual information and outgoing responses is achieved through the perceptual-motor match. The child pays attention to the perceptual data during his active exploration and notes the correspondences between the perceptual data and the exploratory activity. Thus, as he manipulates an object, he watches his hand and relates what he sees to what he feels. Since a body of information has already been started based on exploration, this information becomes the control for the comparison and he learns to see what he has felt.

It is important that the perceptual-motor match be made in this manner with the previous motor-generated information serving as the standard. All perceptual data include certain distortions. Hold a circular disc vertically before your eye. The perceptual data are those of a circle. Now tip the disc slightly. The image cast on the retina of your eye becomes eliptical. Tip the disc somewhat more so that it lies in a plane horizontal to your eye. Now the image on your retina is that of a straight line. The perceptual data were constantly changing and becoming more and more distorted. At all times during this experiment, however, you continued to see a circular disc. You did not see an elipse nor did you see a straight line, even though these data were delivered to you by your sense organ.

In early childhood, during the exploratory phases of learning, you manipulated objects similar to this disc. You observed that as you changed its orientation the object appeared different. Your exploring hand, however, continued to tell you that the object was a circular disc. This exploratory information was used as the standard and you learned to interpret these perceptual distortions in terms of a constant form. The distortions were removed through the perceptual-motor match and perception was corrected to match the motor information.

Held and his associates (5) suggest that if such active exploration does not occur, the distortions presented by perceptual data remain. They investigated the effect of externally produced distortions. By eyeglass lenses and other methods they introduced distortions into visual perception. When their subjects were allowed to actively investigate these perceptions, they rather quickly overcame the distortion and behaved in a manner indicating that they saw in terms of the reality of the objects. When the subjects were prevented from actively investigating and were allowed only to passively observe the phenomena, however, the distortions remained and the subjects continued to make errors in responding to the stimuli. These experiments would suggest that perceptual distortions are corrected only when motor exploration occurs and that their correction results from matching the perceptual data to motor data as a standard.

When the perceptual-motor match is made in the reverse direction, with perceptual data being taken as a standard and motor data altered to fit perceptual data, the child may remain at the mercy of the distortions characterizing perceptual experience. Thus a fifteen-year-old was asked to help lay out a square court on the playground for a game. He stood at a distance where he could observe the entire area and directed other children in where to place the stakes representing the corners of the court. When he had finished, it was noted that the side farthest from him was considerably longer than the line closest to him. He was asked about this but maintained that the two lines were equal. He was then taken to the far end of the playground so that he performed the same task but from this opposite orientation. He now indicated that the line closest to him was too long. Asked to correct it, he committed the same error as before but in the opposite direction.

This youngster showed a failure to establish size constancy. Near objects cast a larger image on the retina than the same object at a greater distance. We learn through locomotor exploration to correct for this distortion so that the man next to us no longer looks like a giant while the man on the opposite curb looks like a pigmy. For such correction, however, the exploratory data must be used as the standard and the perceptual data corrected to match it. A number of observations of the behavior of this youngster indicated that he had matched these variables in the opposite direction, using perception as the standard and matching the response data to it. Such reverse matching left him at the mercy of the distortions characteristic of perceptual data. Such activities as drawing, copying, writing, and the like revealed these distortions influencing his performance.

It is also important that the perceptual-motor match occurs in a wide variety of activities and experiences. As will be pointed out later, there are relationships between perceptions. These relationships can be manipulated without referring them to the organism or the activities of the organism. Comparisons can be made between perceptual data directly. Similarities and differences can be observed without reference to action: as it were, in a disembodied fashion. By this means a rather extensive set of perceptual manipulations can be learned independently of direct response by the organism to these data.

When the perceptual-motor match is limited or spotty, the child may come to live in two different worlds. In one he sees, hears, and experiences perceptually, and in the other he moves and responds. These two worlds may be independent and unrelated, with the result that perceptual information either does not influence behavior or does not influence it properly. Most elementary classrooms contain examples of children who can recognize figures or letters but cannot reproduce them. Many children can readily recite a series of directions but cannot perform the activity described by the directions which they have recited. Many children can read words but cannot reproduce them in writing. It seems possible that in many of these cases the child has developed an inadequate perceptual-motor match so that what he experiences perceptually is not closely related to what he performs responsively. The result is often confusion between the two sets of data with responses unrelated to the information presented.

Ocular Control

A further function of the perceptual-motor match is the control of the external sense organ. This problem is most prominent in the field of vision since the eye is the most mobile of our sense organs. It can be pointed in a large number of directions both horizontally and vertically. The visual information delivered differs—depending on the resulting direction of the gaze. It is necessary that the eye be pointed in the proper direction at any time to deliver the visual information required by the activity in progress.

There are three types of problems involved in the control of the eye. Sometimes there are anatomical difficulties which restrict or confuse the movement of the eye. Muscles may be too short or too long to permit proper movements. This problem is medical in nature and the treatment is usually surgical. Sometimes there are physiological interferences with movement of the eye. Muscles may be weak or poorly functioning. In this event the treatment is orthoptic procedure designed to strengthen and balance the action of the extraocular muscles.

If the anatomical and physiological functions of the organ are adequate, there still remains the problem of learning where to point the eye. The eye must be pointed in a direction which will deliver the proper information. The solution to this problem is based upon knowledge of what the information should be and how to obtain it. It is an educational problem since its major aspects are learning and knowledge. Needless to say, anatomical and physiological problems should be ruled out before a learning approach is taken.

How the child learns to control the eye in the interest of consistent visual information can be illustrated through the development of the familiar eye-hand coordination. In the earliest stages of learning, the child learns to control his hand so that it can give him consistent exploratory data. He then watches his hand as it moves, teaching the eye to follow the hand. He depends upon the information from the hand for consistency and matches the action of the eye to it, so that the visual information is also consistent and matches that from the hand. In this stage, the hand is dominant and guides the eye.

The eye, however, is much more efficient in exploration than the hand. It can range over a greater area and can move much faster and deliver more information per unit of time. Therefore, as soon as control has begun to be established, the eye begins to take over the leading function. Now the eye guides the hand and the hand provides confirming information, or additional information in the event of confusion. The responsibility for consistent information gradually shifts from the hand to the eye.

In the meantime, a consistent body of visual information has been built up. This structured body of visual information comes to serve as a clue to consistency. As a result, the eye can eventually explore on its own without the help of the hand and control is supplied by the body of visual information. Now the hand enters only in the event of extreme complexity or confusion. The eye explores in the same way as the hand did and delivers information which matches that delivered by the hand. At this stage, consistent visual search is possible since the body of information indicates when the sought for data have been encountered, and the consistent pattern of exploration learned from the hand permits an organized search procedure.

Perception

When the child has established a perceptual-motor match so that incoming perceptual information and out-going response information both contribute to the same overall body of knowledge, he can then deal with perceptual data independently. He can compare one perceptual experience with another, noting their similarities and differences. He can isolate one element of a perception and deal with it alone without losing the impression of the whole. He can move from one perception to another and yet maintain an orderly relationship between them.

At this stage in development the child becomes perceptual. He now explores intra- and inter-object relationships through establishment of a body of perceptual information just as he previously did through a combination of perceptual and motor information. He can carry out the same systematic investigation of his environment which he formerly did, but now he need use only perceptual data. Motor information is subsumed, through the perceptual-motor match, by the perceptual data. Overt motor manipulations are necessary only as confirmatory data when the perceptual event is complex or unclear.

When such valid perceptual manipulations are possible, the child can begin to deal with symbolic material. Representations of real perceptual experiences begin to have meaning. He can take a few elements of a real perception, such as those presented in a picture or drawing, and from them construct a valid perceptual experience. He can organize these elements, augmenting or rearranging as necessary, so that a meaningful perception results. Since there is a close relationship between his perceptual information and his response information, the resulting construction is immediately available for problem solving and behavior control.

When perceptual elements can be manipulated validly, vicarious experience is possible. The elements of an experience can be transmitted to the child. He can then combine these elements into a valid perception and gain essentially the same information therefrom that he would have gained from an overt experience. The possibility of such vicarious experience greatly expands the possibilities for increasing his overall body of knowledge.

For vicarious experience to be meaningful to the child, however, he must be able to reorganize the elements into a meaningful articulated experience. He must not continue to deal with elements alone as they are presented to him, but must develop and preserve the relationships between them, for it is the relationships between the elements which constitute the heart of the experience. This aspect of perception has been discussed at length by Strauss (13) in his description of the nature and purpose of form perception. The effectiveness of vicarious experience in the learning of the child is dependent upon the possibility of obtaining the aspects of the form from the transmission of the elements.

As has been pointed out above, form perception and the companion function, figure-ground relationships, grow out of the systematic exploration of the relationships within objects through the contact activities. The perceptual-motor match permits these same functions to be carried out through perceptual manipulations alone without overt motor intervention. When these developments have occurred, purely perceptual manipulations can be carried out in a valid fashion and the resulting observations will give a veridical impression of the environment which can be used with safety and assurance in the solution of problems.

COGNITION

Extensive perceptual manipulations reveal similarities and differences between experiences. Such observation of relationships between perceptions leads to their classification and categorization into clusters or groups. Within such clusters, the relationships can be abstracted and combined into a new whole composed of relationships only. Initial concepts appear to be the result of such perceptual abstractions (14).

Consider your concept of a chair. You have had many perceptual experiences with many different kinds of chairs. There have been hard chairs, soft chairs, wooden chairs, upholstered chairs, metal chairs, etc. Your concept of a chair is a sort of cumulation from all these many perceptual experiences. The cumulation, however, is more than a mere summation. It results from the selection of similar elements among all these many experiences. These similarities are integrated into an abstract whole which is your eventual concept of a chair. There is a sort of "sit-down-ableness" about the content of the concept which cannot directly be described but which constitutes the meaningfulness of the concept. This meaningfulness of the content is the result of the abstraction of relationships from the initial perceptions. It retains its quality of perception, since you remain aware of a perceptual aspect to the whole. On the other hand, it is not identical with any one perception which you have experienced or might experience. Thus initial concepts are abstractions from perceptions.

Such initial concepts are expanded and multiplied by the child until a body of those perceptually based concepts is available to him. These concepts can then be manipulated and combined into more and more abstract concepts in which the perceptual basis is less and less apparent. Thus very abstract conceptions such as "infinity" or "justice" can develop.

The problems of higher cognitive functions such as concept formation and symbolic manipulation are beyond the scope of the present volume. It is important to recognize, however, that the earlier developmental activities of the child lead directly to much more complex operations. In like manner, the efficiency and effectiveness of conceptual manipulations rests on a foundation of perceptual and exploratory bodies of information. Where deficiencies in the latter are found, similar deficiencies in the former are observed. Development is all of one piece and each step is necessary for the next.

DEVELOPMENTAL SEQUENCES

There has been described a sequence of development in the child moving from systematic motor exploration, through perceptual manipulation, to cognitive operations. The child moves step by step through these sequences. When difficulty in learning occurs, one or more steps may be omitted or distorted. In this event it is necessary to determine where the developmental breakdown has occurred and restore the sequence. Special teaching techniques and special training activities may be needed to alleviate the initial difficulty and restore the developmental course. It is such procedures which are described in the present volume with particular reference to the basic abilities underlying perceptual manipulations. Emphasis is laid upon the early stages of development, not because these are the exclusive problems of the child with learning disorders, but because of limitations of space. These early problem areas will be found useful with many children, however, since the interference with learning occurred in many cases at a very early age and hence the interference with development occurred at a very early stage.

Frequently we become concerned with deficiencies in ability displayed by a child in activities appropriate for his chronological age, but we fail to recognize that these apparent deficiencies have their roots in less apparent deficiencies at earlier stages of development. Thus we sometimes treat the symptom rather than the disease. If development could be restored through attention to the problems of earlier stages, the apparent deficiencies in the present activities might be reduced or disappear. We might save much time if, instead of attacking the problem of reading, for example, through more and more reading activities, we insured, through developmental training, that the child possessed the perceptual abilities necessary for the reading task. We may need to build up to reading with some children through more basic learnings before we attack the reading problem itself. What is true of reading, which is a tool skill, is also true of informational learning and problem solving tasks.

It is important to note that the developmental sequences outlined here are a logical succession, not necessarily a chronological succession. Although one step leads to another in the development of higher mental functions, it is not necessarily true that the steps have to be acquired in a strict temporal sequence chronologically. It is the way in which the information is systematized and organized that is important, not the order in which it is acquired. Thus children may be found who have developed facility in perceptual manipulations but have not acquired corresponding ability in motor exploration. They have, in effect, gotten the cart before the horse. Although perceptual activities in such children will probably be distorted and will have limited effect upon the adequacy of their response, it does not follow that a permanent perceptual distortion may be expected. It is quite possible to provide them with a more adequate motor exploratory body of knowledge which they can then integrate with their perceptual knowledge so that the final result does not differ from that of the child who progressed through these functions in the usual order. It does not matter how you acquire the cart and the horse. It only matters how you put them together.

The fact that the developmental process is a logical sequence rather than a chronological one leads to two implications for the training of the child. In the first place, it points out that it is not enough merely to supply information or skills. These data must be organized, and as much or more attention must be given to implementing the organization as is given to imparting the data. Too frequently, training activities are prescribed for children because "every child should be able to do this" or because "it is in the book." Activities are thus provided for themselves alone, not for their contribution to the building of an overall body of knowledge for the child. The result frequently is endless repetition of meaningless activities with which the child quickly becomes bored and which must be forced upon him. When attention is directed toward the logical development of systematic bodies of information, however, activities are prescribed for their immediate contribution to the problems of the child, and selection and evaluation among activities is evident. The child is then motivated toward the training because he can see its relationship to the solution of a problem which is apparent to him now.

The second implication lies in the organization of a program of training. The activities which are prescribed are meaningful and effective in terms of the child's present functioning. Thus motor training activities are one thing to a child who has not developed perceptual facility and another thing to the child who has. The effect of the activity is dependent upon what the child brings to it. The child who has developed perceptual facility will be perceptually oriented and motor activities without a perceptual control will be difficult or impossible for him. On the other hand, activities with a perceptual control will prove easier than might have been expected. Training must start with what the child brings to it. When the child's development is out of logical order, training must be reversed in a similar manner. Systems are built on what is there already. We cannot throw out the old and start in anew. To develop the system, the old must be elaborated and expanded. When development is out of order, training must start there and work down. It cannot start at the bottom and proceed as though it were the child's first learning. He cannot forget what has gone before and training must not forget, but rather adapt, to what has gone before.

Since disparity in development from one area to another is a characteristic symptom of the child with a learning disorder, such alterations of training programs in the light of the child's present status are usually required. It is necessary to determine what the child has been able to build up for himself and use this as a basis for the organization of the training program, altering and modifying it in the light of these disparities. At no time is it possible to approach the training of the child as though nothing had yet happened and a normal developmental history was to be expected. The overall problem of development must be considered and the logical system which is the goal of all training must be evaluated whenever training activities are prescribed. The training will then be prescribed in terms of the overall status of the child relative to the goal of the training.

The activities to be presented in the following chapters are to be considered in this light. Although they are related to the course of development of children, they must be modified and altered to fit the particular developmental problems of the child for whom they are prescribed. A program of training designed to build upon what is found to be strong in the child and augment what is found to be weak must be selected from the list of activities. At no time must the overall problem of a systematic body of information be overlooked. The teacher must continually evaluate and re-evaluate both the program and the child to insure that training does indeed contribute to his welfare.

REFERENCES

1. Coghill, G. E. *Anatomy and the Problem of Behavior.* Cambridge: Cambridge University Press, 1929.

2. Dunsing, J. D. and Kephart, N. C. "Motor Generalizations in Space and Time." In Hellmuth, J. (Ed.) *Learning Disorders, Vol. 1.* Seattle: Special Child Publs., 1965, 77-121.

3. Gesell, A. and Amatruda, C. S. *Developmental Diagnosis.* New York: Paul B. Hoeber, 1941.

4. Godfrey, B. B. and Kephart, N. C. *Movement Patterns and Motor Education.* New York: Appleton-Century-Crofts, in press.

5. Held, R. and Hein, A. "Movement produced stimulation in the development of visually guided behavior." *J. Comp. & Physiol. Psychol.,* 1963, 56, 872-876.

6. Hooker, D. *The Prenatal Origin of Behavior.* Lawrence, Kans.: University of Kansas Press, 1952.

7. Hurlock, E. B. *Child Development.* New York: McGraw-Hill Book Company, 1942.

8. Jersild, A. T. *Child Psychology.* Englewood Cliffs, N. J.: Prentice-Hall, 1954.

9. Kephart, N. C. *The Slow Learner in the Classroom.* Columbus, Ohio: Charles F. Merrill Publishing Company, 1960, 98-114.

10. McCandless, B. R. *Children and Adolescents.* New York: Holt, Rinehart and Winston, 1961.

11. Roach, E. G. and Kephart, N. C. *The Purdue Perceptual-Motor Survey,* Columbus, O.: Charles E. Merrill, Publishing Company, 1966, 4-6.

12. Sherington, C. *The Integrative Action of the Nervous System.* New Haven, Conn.: Yale University Press, 1948.

13. Strauss, A. A. and Kephart, N. C. *Psychopathology and Education of the Brain Injured Child. Volume II.* New York: Grune and Stratton, 1955, 53-61.

14. *Ibid.,* 118-127.

chapter 2

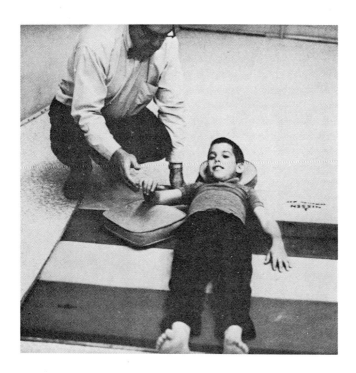

*Movement of a body part without involving other musculature
emphasizes figure-ground.*

How to Structure and
Control Behavior

Before any educational program can result in learning, the child must be capable and willing to participate. Because children with learning difficulties often experience many internal as well as external distractions and interferences, it is often necessary to structure the environment, the task, the materials, and even the child himself. It is also essential that the one who is doing the teaching remains in control of the task and the child at all times until he evidences the ability to structure and control himself.

The ideas presented here are not intended to be the last word on the subject but rather an introduction to the many needs and possibilities. All of them may apply to a group of children at one time or another. Many of them may apply to a particular child. A few will apply to all of the children all of the time.

LEARNING

Keep in mind at all times that a child must "learn to move" before he can "move to learn."

TEACHING

Do not begin teaching on the level where the child is failing. Go back, find the underlying causes of his failure, then help him correct these causes.

LEVELS

You will find it safer and more profitable to begin teaching the slow learner at too low a level rather than too high. By starting too low, the child will experience a series of quick successes and his self-image will be enhanced. If you begin too high, he will learn inadequately, develop splinter skills, or fail as he has so often in the past.

"READINESS"

Think "readiness" until it becomes more important in your curriculum than any academic subject. It is impossible to teach a child that which he is not ready to learn. By the same token, once he is ready to learn, nothing will stop him.

ATTITUDE

Be objective and impersonal at all times. Only then can you recognize the problems for what they are and, together with the child, tackle these problems. You will also find it easier to be firm and even demanding when necessary.

TONE OF VOICE

Use a quiet, authoritative voice. Develop confidence in yourself and the child, and let your voice carry this confidence to the child.

SPEECH

Speak slowly, firmly, and clearly. Keep all directions and commands short, simple, and related to the task. Do not elaborate. The slow learner usually has difficulty sorting out and applying that which is said to him, so each embellishment only adds to his confusion. After the command is given, wait—wait a little longer than you think necessary. Give him time to analyze the command and put it into action. If you feel there is misunderstanding or confusion, repeat the same, simple command again. Remember: He must collect the facts, close the door (so to speak) and correlate them, before he can perform. If he has a motor problem (and most of them do), there will be a second delay as he sorts out the various movements necessary to performance.

Quite often the child will err because he dashes into the task before all directions have been given. To prevent this, insist that the child not move until you have finished the command and occasionally ask him to repeat what you have said before he enters into the task.

CONTROL

Stay in control. As you begin to think of each child at his performance level rather than his age, it will be easier to choose adequate learning materials for him. Once a task is presented (and he can perform it), insist that he follow it through to completion and perform it exactly in the manner you prescribe. Knowing his problems sometimes better than we know them, the child will often vary or rearrange the task slightly to avoid his learning difficulties. If, however, he is permitted to continue in this manner, very little learning will take place. If he suggests a variation, you might say, "Okay, just as soon as you do it this way, we will try your way." In other words, do not let the child gain control of the learning activity.

Remember that you are to structure all tasks and give the commands. The child faced with a difficult situation will use many methods to avoid a task he thinks he might fail. He may try to make minor changes, verbalize about anything but the task before him, resist, act foolish, throw a tantrum, disturb others, giggle, develop aches and pains, etc., etc., etc. Stop these overtures, or if this is momentarily impossible, work right through them or, in case of the verbalization, direct it toward the task.

Many of the above behaviorisms are self defeating, disruptive to training, and impossible to terminate through outside negative reinforcement. Swatting, reasoning, or pressure from other children seem only to increase the behaviors. Thus the behavior itself must become inherently punishing to the child. To accomplish this, the child must be made to "over-do" the behavioral sequence in question.

Thus the child who hits, kicks, throws a tantrum, or uses other methods of avoiding performance can best be dealt with by making his behaviorism more uncomfortable than proper performance. If he kicks, sit him on the floor, hold him in place, and insist that he kick until you and he are exhausted. If he bites, insist that he bite on a piece of hard rubber or other harmless but uncomfortable substance. If he throws a tantrum with kicking, striking, and yelling, grasp him firmly and tell him to go ahead and "blow." If he stops, tell him to yell some more but add, "When you are finished yelling, you will perform the task." Thus even the control of overt behavior can be achieved through motor performance. It works because it attacks the problem in two ways. It makes task performance more comfortable than non-performance, and it drains off excess motor energy.

TASKS

If the given task proves too difficult, restructure it; then train toward it. Keep in mind the three levels of performance and try to present tasks that are challenging to the child. If occasionally you err and present a task that is too difficult and therefore frustrating, do not remove the task but quickly restructure it, thus simplifying it to the level where the child can perform. Then put it away for a few weeks or months while you present tasks at a lower performance level, thus preparing him to achieve the original task at a later date.

We advocate simplifying the task to let the child experience some feeling of success, but even more important to let him know that the resistance brought on by frustration will not automatically make a task go away. For, if the child finds this to be true, he often shows signs of frustration each time a task requires him to really work to succeed.

An example of simplifying the task was the teacher whose pupil had learned to "draw" a square. She then presented him with a peg board and pegs, presuming that he was aware of all the elements of squareness, and said, "Make a square." The child looked baffled but started placing pegs in a row and continued to the end of the board and stopped. The teacher said, "No, that is a line. Make a square." Again, the same result. This continued until both teacher and pupil were frustrated and the child, in tears, pushed the board off the table. Being a wise teacher, she had the child pick up the pieces, thus giving herself time to think. Suddenly she realized that drawing a square and constructing one from tiny elements that must be arranged in a certain pattern of lines and angles were not equal tasks. Once the board and pegs were back on the table, she placed the four corner pegs and instructed the child to fill in the lines between the goals, thus making a square. She then spent the next few weeks having the children move along form outlines with their bodies as well as their hands. She had them construct forms using a large variety of media: their bodies, large boards, tongue depressors, blocks, etc. They matched forms and explored them with their hands and fingers. When finally they returned to the peg board, the task was executed with aplomb and pride, yet no training on the peg board had been done.

COMMANDS

Quite often it is necessary for more than one person to work with a rebellious or extremely uncoordinated child, but only one should give commands. The second person should only supply an extra pair of hands. If there is disagreement as to how the task should be performed, discuss it after the work session, not in front of the child. Parents often encounter this difficulty. While they enter into a heated or lengthy discussion as to how it should be done, the child escapes, thus avoiding the task he didn't want to perform in the first place, and no learning takes place. Even if he is returned to the task, how can you possibly convey to him the feeling of confident expectancy when the adults involved are not in agreement.

ORIENTATION

Always remain task oriented. If the child resists, do not scold him for being naughty; direct him back to the task. Your attitude should say, "You can do it," and "I'm going to see that you do."

MOVES

Learn to anticipate the child's abortive and resistive moves before he makes them. So often the child is not aware of the origin of the move, or if he is aware he does not know how to control it; therefore, all punishment after the fact is useless. The child who jumps out of his chair and leaves the task can be brought back a hundred times; still he wins a hundred times. Only if you anticipate what comes before his dash for freedom can you move in and prevent it at it's source. Then you begin to win: first, because you make the child aware of the initial move; and second, because now he knows that he can learn to control it and often does so rather quickly.

A favorite story is of a family who nearly quit going to church as a family because they had been tackling such a problem at the wrong end. It was during the era when many well-dressed ladies were wearing hats with a tall feather to one side—a tall feather that moved most distractingly with each little breath of air. The family had a young daughter who simply could not resist such feathers, and no matter where they sat in church, a plume-hatted lady seemed to find her way into the seat just ahead of them. And each Sunday the wearer managed to lose her hat. Sometime during the church service the child fixated on the feather and automatically her hand shot forward. The next moment the feather, hat and all, was in her hands, instead of on the lady's head. The child had been spanked, threatened, kept home once or twice, etc., etc., but nothing seemed to help. Finally the mother analyzed the whole problem and noted that the child always reached with her right hand. The next Sunday she sat at the child's right side and found that she could interpret a tensing of the right shoulder as the move that preceded the thrust of the arm. The mother thus solved her problem by leaving her left hand free to use as a slide bolt that quickly slid in front of her young daughter's arm just as it started to move forward. As the two collided, the child became aware of just what it was that Mother wanted her to stop, and after a few Sundays this maneuver was no longer necessary.

CONCENTRATION

Do not move the child too quickly from one task to another. When the child is concentrating on a task, items of information pertinent to that task are grouped or integrated into the structure of the task as a whole.

At that moment the child can move about at will within the cluster of acts or ideas pertinent to the task. But the very processing that holds these items together prevents him from moving or acting outside of the cluster.

If someone introduces a new and unrelated stimulus, the child is incapable of dropping the task in which he is involved at the moment and therefore he cannot enter into the new task. If the person presenting the new task insists and pressures the child, he will react in one of several ways:

a. If he is completely involved in his present task, he may not *be aware* of the new stimulus.

b. He may be aware of it, but because it makes no sense to him, he will *ignore it.*

c. He may *deliberately shut it and you out,* not only because the new task makes no sense to him, but also because attending to you causes confusion in the present task. If at this point you pressure or demand, the child will rebel because he honestly does not understand what you are asking of him.

d. He may *integrate* the *new stimulus* into his present structure. To do this he will probably *distort the stimulus* that was presented, taking out, extracting from the total stimulus those parts that can readily be integrated.

Example: Mother says, "Johnny, tell Grandma who you are going to see at church tomorrow." The obvious answer is Mr. Hebb, the Sunday school teacher, of whom Johnny is terribly fond and of whom he is constantly talking. But at the moment Johnny is completely involved with watching the garbage truck and the men emptying the garbage cans; mother repeats her question, demanding an answer. Johnny catches the inference that he is to tell Grandma about somebody so he answers, "The garbage man." Mother is horrified, scolds a little, so Johnny starts name guessing, names his teachers, friends, etc., hoping to hit on the right one. If success is too long in coming, *he blows.*

We are more apt to err in this fashion with the hypo-active child, for so much of his doing is passive while the normal child is busy moving about. To the on-looker, he may seem to be doing nothing when he really may be intensely involved; with his limited motor-output he may be fully involved although little action is seen.

The normal child who finds himself in this situation says, "Wait a minute," and we wait, for we know that he is eventually going to obey us. So often the hypo-active child either cannot say "Wait" or is too involved to say it. Even when he does say "Wait," we are not as willing to do so because we can never be sure that he is going to obey us anyway. So we demand and he explodes. He cannot cope with the problem intellectually, so he reverts to a lower level and responds emotionally.

STABILITY

Try not to interfere with the child's temporal stability. The child may be living without an adequate internal time structure. Because he cannot structure time for himself, he becomes a stickler for routine. He depends on the routine to structure his day. Any change, even a slight one, upsets him terribly.

If you present a task in the place of or out of rhythm with whatever the child is using to structure his time, he is suddenly thrust into an unstructured temporal situation and is uncomfortable and sometimes frightened; therefore, he rejects it.

If you take him from an unfinished task, by his standards it remains dangling. It has no end and there is an abyss.

When you attempt to thrust him immediately into a new activity which has no structured beginning or end (all you have said is "Come and do"), he becomes lost and uncomfortable and resists.

DISTRACTION

Keep the child's eyes on the task. If the child cannot keep his eyes on the task, call him back repeatedly. Do not scold or verbalize all the reasons why he should be looking; rather, tap the table or desk top to call him back. If you talk about it, his eyes will automatically go to the area that is creating the greatest distraction at the moment—your mouth.

"NO"

Use the word "no" sparingly. Do not say "no" unless you intend to carry through and see to it that the child obeys. If you say "no" today, be sure that similar actions will bring forth a forceful "no" with the same repercussions an hour later, tomorrow, or next week.

Too often parents and teachers say, "No, no, Johnny—don't do that," and then each goes on doing as he was. The adult feels that he has conveyed to the child the idea that the activity is not acceptable. Too often, however, the reverse is true. The word "no" loses all its significance to the child when it is not enforced. So think twice before you say "no." Once you have said it, be prepared to stop whatever you may be doing to enforce the word "no."

RELAXATION

Teach the child to relax. Any child who must tense his whole body before he can perform simple motor or perceptual tasks receives inadequate information from the key movements and, therefore, performs inadequately. Once you have performance upon command, the next important goal is performance out of relaxation.

Consider the child who, in order to pull the eyes into focus to read, tenses his whole body. Such a child concentrates so completely on the act of reading that nothing is left to concentrate on content. He reads fluently; then someone asks the wrong question—"What did you read?" He has no idea.

Or simpler still, the child who has never moved an arm without tensing every muscle in his body—he is never really sure when or how the arm will move. Each time he uses it he receives messages from every area of his body, never one clear, distinct message from that arm. So he has very little information upon which to build an adequate movement pattern. Such a child does not know what it is to relax; therefore, a verbal suggestion will not suffice. He will need to feel relaxation in at least a portion of his body and recognize it for what it is before he can learn to relax the whole body.

REACTIONS

Mother—Dad—Teacher: Relax. The child quickly senses your tensions and reacts adversely to them. Rome wasn't built in a day. Once you find the child's performance level and can present learning tasks at that level, progress will be faster—but don't expect the impossible. Consider how much progress would be made by a normal child and then be thankful if you come anywhere near that goal. To expect more is foolhardy and will certainly result in frustration for all concerned.

SENSE OF HUMOR

Develop a sense of humor. There will be times when to relieve the buildup of tensions you will need to laugh or cry, and laughter is the better medicine.

section 2

chapter 3

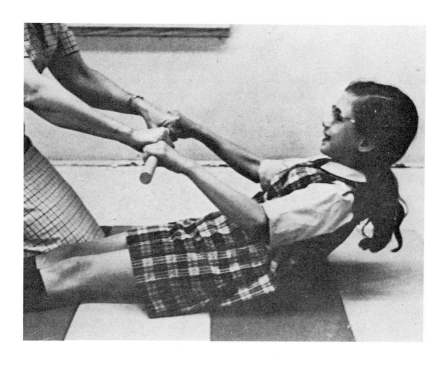

Adequate development of motor response showing cephalo-caudal direction.

Procedures for Evaluation

The Purdue Perceptual-Motor Survey* offers a convenient procedure for evaluating motor performance and its relation to perceptual awareness. This scale presents activities designed to elicit behavior indicative of abilities in the area of balance and posture, body image and differentiation, perceptual-motor matching, ocular control, and form perception. The survey consists of twenty-two observations. The child's performance on each of these items is compared to standardized descriptions of behavior, and that description most nearly fitting the observed performance is selected. Rating scores are assigned to each standard description in terms of its reflection of adequacy in perceptual-motor behavior. When the appropriate description has been selected, the accompaning rating score is credited. Thus numerical scores indicative of adequacy of behavior are obtained.

The record form provides for graphic entry of scores. The resulting profile is used to aid in determining the area or areas in which intensive training should be concentrated. It is desirable that these standardized observations be supplemented by clinical observations of the examiner.

Until you develop a "clinical eye" for observing behavior in the child's performance on the Perceptual-Motor Survey and to help you develop that clinical eye, the following observation lists have been designed. Their

---

*Eugene G. Roach and Newell C. Kephart, *The Purdue Perceptual-Motor Survey* (Columbus, Ohio: Charles E. Merrill Publishing Company, 1966).

use will not only enhance your ability to observe the items more discretely, but will also make it easier to prepare training activities better suited to the child's needs. As you observe and analyze the child's performance, look for a pattern of difficulties and try to relate that which is observed to the overall problem. Thus you will be better able to concentrate on those pertinent to the child's learning difficulties.

In this way the resulting training program will not be too diversified nor too limited, i.e. you will not attempt to put the child through all the training activities. Neither will you pick a specific item that the child has failed and spend hours or weeks trying to correct it. Example: If a child always carries his arms bent at the elbow with his hands up and his upper arm extended out slightly from the body in order to maintain balance or catch himself if he sways too far to the side, it would be fruitless to concentrate on arm extension unless the balance problem was corrected first or at least simultaneously.

You will find the observation lists particularly helpful: first, for the younger child, 3 through 5 years, who would not be expected to perform many of the PMS items; second, for the older child with gross basic problems who scores all No. 1's or 0's; third, for the older child who seemingly performs all items well but leaves you with the feeling that there is something amiss, something you just can't put your finger on or cannot analyze. The third type of child is usually one who has developed a series of "splinter skills" or one who has been trained in the PMS items. Of the latter: the therapists at the Achievement Center for Children often speak jokingly of the "Angels" reflex. They are referring to the child who, when asked to lie on his back or on the floor, starts doing "Angels in the Snow" movements the moment the therapist points at a limb and before she has time to give a command. If a statement on the observation lists applies to the child being observed, place a check mark in the box at the end of the statement. If the statement does not apply, no mark is made. No scoring is necessary. Summarize the checked items to determine the child's motor and visual-motor deficits.*

---

*Separate checklists, including both the OBSERVATIONS OF BASIC MOTOR MOVEMENTS and OBSERVATIONS OF VISUAL MOTOR MOVEMENTS lists, are available in quantities of 20 forms per package from Charles E. Merrill Publishing Company, 1300 Alum Creek Drive, Columbus, Ohio (code number 9566).

OBSERVATIONS OF BASIC MOTOR MOVEMENTS

MOVEMENTS AND POINTS TO OBSERVE	COMMENTS

I. DIFFERENTIATION

A. *Head Control* (child on his back on the floor)

1. Observe head position as child pulls up to sitting position. Hold a pole (broomstick) for the child to pull on. Head should lift easily and first, shoulders should follow. Note if:

   a. Shoulders tense and lift first with head lagging behind. ☐

   b. Head is "tied into" the shoulders and all lift as a unit. ☐

2. Observe child's ability to lift only the head while lying on back and on stomach. Can he easily lift his head and look about? Note if:

   a. It is necessary to tense the whole body first. ☐

   b. There is tension in other limbs. ☐

   c. Child is unable to lift or move head. ☐

B. *Trunk Differentiation* (child on his stomach or back as required)

1. Can the child differentiate at the waistline? Can he lift knees and

MOVEMENTS AND POINTS TO OBSERVE	COMMENTS

move them from side to side touching floor while keeping shoulders on the mat? Can he pivot the upper trunk without moving hips and legs? (The pivoting can be done by swaying back and forth or on the stomach; the elbows or hands can be used to propel the upper trunk back and forth in a semicircle.) Note if:

a. Child cannot move upper trunk without involving or moving lower trunk. ☐

b. Child cannot move lower trunk without involving or moving upper trunk. ☐

2. Can the child differentiate the four quadrants of the trunk? Can he enervate and move a shoulder or hip without involving other parts of the body? (Have the child try a variety of hip and shoulder movements. Note if:

a. To move one leg at the hip the other leg becomes involved and moves also. ☐

b. To move one arm at the shoulder the other shoulder, the head, or a leg becomes involved in the movement. ☐

c. A quadrant can be moved alone but the remainder of the body tenses. ☐

3. Since true differentiation presupposes that differentiated parts can also be used in combination, it is

MOVEMENTS AND POINTS TO OBSERVE	COMMENTS

well to check and see if the child can move parts of the body simultaneously. Note if:

a. The thrust or movement is not truly bilateral— that is, if one side has more thrust or seems to lead the other.
Bilateral hip thrust. ☐

Bilateral shoulder thrust. ☐

b. Upper trunk cannot move without involving the lower trunk, and reverse. ☐

4. Simultaneous unilateral movement of shoulders and hips can also be explored and observations made as in B.3. above.

a. Right shoulder and hip. ☐

b. Left shoulder and hip. ☐

C. *Limb Differentiation* (child on stomach or back as required)

1. Requires a variety of arm and leg movements in all directions close to the body and in full extension. (Give the child a goal to reach toward or follow with hand or foot.) Note if:

a. The child can move his hands into tasks only if the upper arms are kept close to the body and all movement comes from the elbows. ☐

MOVEMENTS AND POINTS TO OBSERVE   COMMENTS

b. He uses a fully extended arm with little or no elbow movements. ☐

c. Movements back and forth between the two extremes are rigid, jerky, and uncontrolled. ☐

d. There are areas in which the limb cannot move with ease. ☐

e. The child cannot cross the "midline" of his body without moving the head or trunk. ☐

f. The child changes hand or foot at the midline or acts as if he would like to do so. ☐

If the child's problem is basically one of inadequate differentiation it will be quite evident at this point. If, however, he has passed the above tests but has failed such items as angels and jumping on the PMS, it would suggest that differentiation is hampered by a lack of adequate balance or that the child has not learned to use the differentiated parts in combination.

The following items are to help pinpoint such problems:

II. BALANCE AND COORDINATED DIFFEREN-
TIATION

A. *Changing Positions*

1. Observe how the child goes from:

a. Standing to sitting.
b. Standing to lying down.

MOVEMENTS AND POINTS TO OBSERVE	COMMENTS

     c. From prone to standing.
     d. From supine to standing.
     e. Standing to squatting and up again.

  2. Note if:

     a. Movements are non-differentiated. ☐

     b. The child pushes up bilaterally and flops down the same way. ☐

     c. The child moves very quickly and cannot perform slowly on command without losing his balance or control of the movements. ☐

     d. The child cannot vary the task but must perform the one and only way he knows. ☐

B. *Sitting*

  1. Observe the child's balance as he sits on the floor, in a chair, at a desk or table. Sitting on the floor, note if:

     a. He cannot sit erect with the legs extended. ☐

     b. He folds his legs back at the knees and sits between his own legs for balance. (The legs in a ＼ᴖ／ position.) ☐

     c. The body and arms are rigid rather than relaxed. ☐

MOVEMENTS AND POINTS TO OBSERVE	COMMENTS

2. Sitting in a chair or at a desk. Note if:

   a. The child slumps. ☐

   b. He must hold on. ☐

   c. He constantly leans on one arm for support. ☐

   d. There is frequent shifting, squirming, or readjusting of weight mass. ☐

C. *Standing*

1. Observe the child's balance as he stands. Note if:

   a. The child cannot stand still for 30 to 60 seconds without loosing his balance. ☐

   b. There is quite a lot of swaying from side to side or fore and aft. ☐

   c. There are shifts of weight from one side to the other. ☐

   d. All the weight is placed on one leg. ☐

   e. The feet are set far apart to give a wide base for balance. ☐

   f. He cannot sway purposefully from side to side and fore and aft while the feet remain in one spot. ☐

   g. The purposeful swaying is not rhythmic. ☐

MOVEMENTS AND POINTS TO OBSERVE	COMMENTS

2. Observe whether the child can stand for several seconds on each foot. Note if:
   a. Balance is extremely difficult. □
   b. He ties the "up" leg in against the standing leg. □
   c. He can balance on one foot, but not the other. □
   d. He cannot maintain balance for more than 1 or 2 seconds. □

D. *Locomotion*

1. Observe the patterns of differentiation as the child crawls *across the floor on his stomach.* With a younger child it may be necessary for the therapist to place her hand on the child's back or hip until he gets the feel of what is expected of him. The older child can be told to imitate the Marines going under a barbed wire barricade or across a battle field with bullets flying over his head. Even older boys will accept the task when presented this way. The front of the trunk should be flat on the floor and only the limbs should propel the body forward. Note if:
   a. The child has difficulty initiating movement. □
   b. The child has difficulty maintaining movement. □
   c. One or two limbs are not incorporated into the movement. □

MOVEMENTS AND POINTS TO OBSERVE   COMMENTS

---

    d. The movement is a flop-
ping from side to side
with the trunk rather than
differentiated pulling and
pushing with the arms and
legs. ☐

    e. There is no maintenance
of a pattern, just a series
of uncoordinated move-
ments. ☐

    f. He becomes so involved
in the movements that he
looses sight of the goal. ☐

2. Observe the child's patterns of differentiation as he creeps toward a
target *on his hands and knees.* Note
if:

    a. He cannot keep his eyes
on the target as he ap-
proaches it. ☐

    b. He keeps his eyes on the
target but loses the movement pattern in doing so. ☐

    c. There is no pattern to
his movements. ☐

    d. He cannot maintain the
movement when varia-
tions are introduced. *Example*: Pushing a large
block with both hands,
pushing a smaller block
with one hand. ☐

    e. He can maintain the pat-
tern only at one speed. ☐

E. *Walking and Running*
   Observe the child as he walks and runs
about the room.

MOVEMENTS AND POINTS TO OBSERVE	COMMENTS

1. *Forward*—note if:

   a. The trunk is not erect. ☐
   b. The hands are not swing- ☐
      ing at his side.
   c. The legs move rigidly
      from the hips or are held
      rigidly in place at the hips
      and move only from the ☐
      knee.
   d. The feet shuffle along not ☐
      leaving the floor.
   e. He has difficulty starting ☐
      or stopping.
   f. He cannot vary the speed
      on command while mov- ☐
      ing.
   g. He simply sways the body
      from side to side when
      moving thus lifting a leg
      or foot as the weight pro- ☐
      pels it forward.
   h. He can vary the speed
      but stops or hesitates at ☐
      each change.
   i. He cannot start and stop ☐
      on command.
   j. His concentration on the
      movements interferes ☐
      with assigned tasks.

2. *Other Directions*
   Can the child walk sideways or
   backwards on command or imitating? Note if:

   a. There is difficulty initiat- ☐
      ing the movement.
   b. There is difficulty main-
      taining the movement or ☐
      the direction.

MOVEMENTS AND POINTS TO OBSERVE   COMMENTS

c. He shuffles. ☐
d. When going sideways he crosses one leg over the other (cannot maintain lead with one foot). ☐
e. He cannot vary the speed. ☐
f. He cannot start or stop on command. ☐
g. He cannot move in a straight line. ☐

F. *Galloping* (forerunner of the skip)

1. Have the child gallop across the floor leading with one foot then the other. Note if:

a. He cannot gallop. ☐
b. He has difficulty initiating or stopping. ☐
c. He cannot maintain. ☐
d. He can perform with one foot leading but not the other. ☐
e. Movements are rigid and very little differentiation is seen. ☐

G. *Gliding* (essential to hip differentiation)

1. Have the child glide (move sideways across the floor, lifting and stepping with the lead foot, hop-

MOVEMENTS AND POINTS TO OBSERVE   COMMENTS

---

ping lightly on the other) across
the floor. Note if:

a. He cannot perform.   ☐
b. He has difficulty initiat-   ☐
   ing or stopping.
c. He cannot maintain.
d. He can perform with one
   foot leading but not the   ☐
   other.
e. The movements are rigid
   and very little differentia-   ☐
   tion is seen.

OBSERVATIONS OF VISUAL MOTOR MOVEMENTS

I. FIXATIONS WITH REACH, GRASP, AND RELEASE

These activities are designed to check the child's ability to make the perceptual-motor match, so necessary to learning.

The point is to see whether the child can fixate on an object and maintain the fixation until his hand reaches and grasps it; whether he can maintain this fixation while a purposeful act is performed, such as fixating on a container until the hand releases the object into the container. Unless the child can maintain visual contact with the hand as it performs the task, the perceptual-motor match is not adequate.

As the child reaches and grasps, observe his grasping technique. An inferior grasp can indicate motor problems in the arm and hand, a perceptual problem, or both. Perceptual because, if the child does not look as he grasps, he will have to continue to use a palmar sweep or miss that for which he reaches.

Materials needed:

1. Large objects to be placed into a large container (blocks, etc. into a box).
2. Small objects to be placed into a small container (buttons, pegs, etc. into a bottle).

The child is to take each object as it is presented to him and then place it in the container. Vary the point of presentation and move the container often during the observation period, otherwise the child is apt to memorize the position and, therefore, not need to keep his eyes on the task.

Keep all goals within arm's reach, otherwise it is difficult to know whether the body involvement is due to lack of differentiation or a necessity for reaching the target.

OBSERVATIONS   COMMENTS

1. Is there an inconsistent use of hands? ☐

2. If not, does he change hands to avoid crossing the midline? ☐

3. Does the child resist using one of his hands? Which one? ☐

4. Does he tilt his head, possibly occluding one eye? Which eye? ☐

5. Is there just one area where the child performs most adequately and uses eyes and hands simultaneously? ☐

   (This area will serve as a starting point when training is introduced.)

6. Does he seemingly look at the object or target, then over- or under-reach? (The problem may be lack of hand control or lack of perceptual orientation.) ☐

7. Is there extreme difficulty or inability to grasp or release? ☐

If the child has difficulty releasing into a container, have him place the object in your hand or on the table.

If he has difficulty grasping, present objects for him to reach out and touch, and observe the reach, touch, and release.

It may be necessary to use sound making gadgets or other interesting objects to hold his attention (a bell, twirling sparkler, rattle, tambourine, etc.).

OBSERVATIONS   COMMENTS

A. *Reaching*

   1. Is the reach unusually

      fast?   ☐

      slow?   ☐

      uncontrolled?   ☐

   2. Does the child lean forward with
      the whole body rather than   ☐
      reaching out with the arm?

   3. When reaching to full extension,
      does the child have difficulty   ☐
      contacting the object?

      or fail to reach the object?   ☐

   4. Does the child turn or sway the
      body when the hand and eyes   ☐
      are required to cross the midline?

   5. Is it necessary to hold the child
      in place to prevent the turning   ☐
      and swaying?

   6. Does holding in place interfere   ☐
      with performance?

   7. Does the child have difficulty
      when required to reach out and   ☐
      back repeatedly?

   8. Are there areas where the child
      has difficulty reaching and per-   ☐
      forming?

B. *Grasping*

   1. Is the type of grasp inadequate   ☐
      for the task?

OBSERVATIONS   COMMENTS

2. Is there tension in the grasping hand or the unused digits? ☐

3. Is there lack of tonus in the grasping hand or unused digits? ☐

4. Does the child locate the objects with his eyes, begin the approach with the hand, then turn the eyes away before the hand contacts the objects? ☐

C. *Releasing*

1. Does the child fail to keep his eyes on the container until the object is released? ☐

2. Does he locate the container with his eyes, then look away as the hand approaches, using hand or finger to locate the container tactually before releasing? ☐

3. Is the release tense and uncontrolled? ☐

4. Does he have difficulty releasing the object? ☐

5. Does he consistently toss, throw, or drop the object? ☐

   (Is the above an indication of inability to release or a behavior problem?)

6. Does he release too soon? ☐

7. Does he release too late? ☐

II. PURSUITS

Move a target before the child's eyes as in the Perceptual-Motor Survey. Require the child to follow the target with his eyes and his hand. (Have him point at the target with the finger approximately one inch from the target.) The arm should be extended and relaxed, not resting on elbow on the table. When checking reaching movements, move the target in near-to-far positions, as well as vertical, horizontal, etc.

Begin the task with the target moving back and forth across the midline of the child's body. If there are indications of extreme difficulty due to inability to make the crossover, then simplify the task by moving the target from the midline (nose area) out into the various areas of the periphery. Results will indicate where to begin training.

To perform adequately, the eyes and hands should move in unison into all areas within the child's reach and the movements should be smooth, synchronous, and controlled.

OBSERVATIONS   COMMENTS

Lack of visual motor match is indicated
if:

1. The eye movements are less adequate when the hand is involved. ☐

2. The hand has difficulty following the target. ☐

3. The pointed finger and the eyes never seem to be in exactly the same place at the same time. ☐

4. The child anticipates the movements and moves hands and eyes in the general direction of the moving target, but does not actually follow it. ☐

5. Hand, eyes, or both fail to stop when target stops. ☐

OBSERVATIONS   COMMENTS

6. Target is lost by hand or eyes, or both when midline is crossed. ☐

7. There is a break or hesitation at the midline, then eyes and hand continue to move in the correct direction, sometimes catching up with the target, sometimes overshooting. ☐

8. The child rejects the task after the first or second try by shutting his eyes, refusing to look or point at the target. ☐

9. The child follows rather well by tensing his whole body to perform but performance breaks down if movement is repeated 4 or 5 times. ☐

If the child's balance problem is such that it interferes with performance, more adequate observations can be made if the child is anchored in his chair with a seat belt or placed on his back on a mat or table.

Further observations can be made at the chalkboard. If the child's performance level is so low that it cannot be assessed by the items on the Perceptual-Motor Survey, ask the child to scribble or draw and observe his body and arm movements, his grasp and release of the chalk, and his eye-hand coordination as he performs.

GUIDELINES FOR SELF-HELP AND MOTOR DEVELOPMENT

When working with the child with learning difficulties, we sometimes fail because we do not have a good overview of how the normal child grows, develops, and moves.

We know from observing "normal children" that there are no two alike in the speed or extent of their motor learning. Children in the regular classroom or in a single family vary considerably in how soon they sit, talk, walk, draw, etc. Children with learning disabilities show more extreme rates of development both fast and slow, and they often do not follow the sequential growth and development patterns.

This information is presented for parents, teachers, and others concerned with the slow learning child. It will serve only to help estimate the degree of motor retardation present in a child, and to aid in understanding the normal sequence of physical development*

AGE	ACCOMPLISHMENTS INVOLVING MOTOR SKILLS
Birth	Little head control. Grasp is a reflex action. Release not possible.
1 Month	Reacts with mass motor activity to any stimulation. Hands kept fisted. Startles in response to sudden loud noises.
2 Months	Can hold up head for several seconds. Vigorous movements in bath. May smile when caressed. Some babbling.
3 Months	If a child is held erect, head wobbles slightly. Holds toy for short time. Inspects hands as he moves them about. Picks at clothing. Coos and chuckles.
4 Months	Rotates head from side to side while lying on back. Can hold head steadily erect if supported in a sitting position. Moves fingers; scratches. Reaches for toy and grasps it. Turns head toward a sound. Plays with hands or a rattle.

*Adapted from: Arnold Gesel, *et al, The First Five Years of Life* (New York: Harper & Row, Publishers, 1940), 65-107.

5 Months	Can momentarily support large fraction of his weight in standing position. Can roll over by rotating upper part of the body, flexing hips, and throwing leg to same side. Rolls from his back to face-down position.
6 Months	Holds head erect easily, and can rotate it. Supports self on outstretched arms. Can grasp rattle and transfer it from hand to hand. Fingers reflections in a mirror.
7 Months	Momentarily can hold trunk erect in a sitting position. Assumes crawl position with weight supported on one or both arms. Dances and bounces when held in upright position. Grasps rattle well with both hands. May inadvertently drop object during hand-to-hand transfer. Reaches out for people.
8 Months	Can support entire body weight on feet for short intervals. Pivots about by using arms. Bangs spoon on table in imitation.
9 Months	Can hold trunk erect indefinitely in sitting position. Can lean forward and regain sitting position. Can stand on toes. Assumes creeping position on hands and knees. Pokes objects using an index finger.
10 Months	Can pull self to knees and can stand with support. May attempt to wave "bye bye." Drinks from cup when assisted.
11 Months	Can go from sitting to face-down to sitting position. Intentional finger release begins.
12 Months	Can lower self from standing to sitting by holding onto crib rails, chair, or other support. Cruises or walks about using support. Reaches for objects, not only to grasp them, but also to use them. Rolls or throws ball rolled to him. May attempt to feed self awkwardly.
13 Months	Can creep on hands and knees. Has reached good proficiency in releasing or dropping objects.
15 Months	Can stand quite independently. Climbs stairs if one hand is held. Opens and closes small boxes.

18 Months	Good sitting balance. Can sit without support. Can get into high chair with difficulty, turn around, and sit down. In high chair, if he reaches for object, always places opposite hand on table to balance self. Stands with both feet on floor. Toddles about, but turns around poorly. Reaches almost automatically for near objects. Grasps small object with wide open hand. Opens drawers. Climbs onto chairs and beds. Throws ball. Brings toys on request. Feeds self. Attempts to put on clothing but without success.
20 Months	Stands on one foot with help.
21 Months	Begins to run. Can walk up flight of three steps alone. Kicks large balls. Scribbles spontaneously.
24 Months	Picks up objects from floor. Holds objects without dropping them. May step over chair in seating himself. Walks steadily if unhurried. Can imitate clapping, raising arms over head, revolving hands. Begins to hold crayon with fingers. Can turn pages singly.
3 Years	Stands with little conscious effort. Stands on one foot momentarily without support. Can walk and run on toes, walk in straight line, and jump off floor with feet together. Can catch large ball with arms extended stiffly. Can ride tricycle with great dexterity. Can sit well, but reaches out somewhat awkwardly. Can pick up small objects with ease. Handles crayons like an adult. Unbuttons front and side buttons of clothes, but has great difficulty in buttoning.
4 Years	Carries cup of water without spilling. Takes pleasure in stunts, i.e., whirling, swinging, somersaulting. Can duckwalk. Can catch ball, but uses arms more than hands in receiving the ball. Grasps cube neatly with thumb and middle finger, and smaller objects well with thumb and index finger. Can adjust grasp to brush teeth.
5 Years	Keen sense of balance. Marches well in time to music. Less cautious in movements than four-year-old. Performs with greater speed, precision, and confidence than

four-year-old. Shows great precision in use of tools (toothbrush, silverware, pencil). Can tie bow knot. Manipulates buttons well. Can lace shoes and can build cube tower well.

6 Years   Can stand on each foot alternately with eyes closed. Can bow gracefully. Reaches well. Movements of head, trunk, and arms are smoothly synchronized. Uses great care in building cube tower, and checks frequently on alignment.

section 3

chapter 4

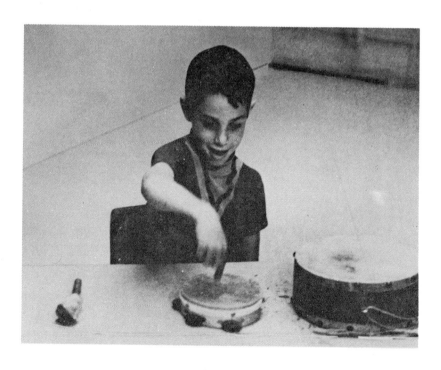

Sound discrimination is a forerunner of speech and language discrimination.

Learning to Listen[*]

By Sylvia B. Kottler

It may seem strange to include a chapter on listening in a series on motoric aids to learning, but as you work through the activities, you will quickly come to the realization that there are two basic and legitimate reasons for doing so.

First of all, listening is a learned process and it is learned in conjunction with movements. In the beginning, the child startles at quick or loud sounds and seems to ignore others. A little later he becomes aware of more sounds and moves or "cocks" his head slightly to localize the sound, then turns the head to locate the source with his eyes. As the child develops more movement patterns, he moves in the direction of a sound to locate and identify it. Without these movements, sound would remain meaningless to the child.

Secondly, even without the motor component, training in the art of listening is necessary. Unless a child learns to listen and attend to the activities in his environment, he cannot and will not learn maximally from that environment.

The normal development of auditory attention depends upon a number of biological and environmental factors: an adequate hearing mechanism; an ability to attend, i.e. to select "foreground" sounds from the

---

*Much of this chapter has been adapted from a paper, "Learning to Listen II," prepared by Sylvia Kottler, Speech Pathologist, Achievement Center for Children, Purdue University.

general background of noise; and an ability to decode the auditory signal, which requires the child to match efficiently and promptly the incoming auditory impression with previously stored inner language experience.

In the actual development of spoken language, there is a comparatively long time-lag between learning to listen and learning to talk. Ordinarily, the infant learns to listen in close mother-proximity, in "homely" or familiar situations that are repeated frequently. When the infant fails to receive this kind of stimulation early, the environmental situation is changed by the time he is ready. He is more mobile, and his mother's voice is heard from a greater distance and probably not as often. He attends to other stimuli instead. It is, therefore, important to keep in mind the child's auditory-spatial world. Clinical tests have demonstrated that beyond five or six feet very young children do not attend auditorally. With the child who is not a good listener, admonishing or telling him to pay attention is rarely enough. Instead, if you want to capture his attention, stop what you are doing, make sure that he looks directly at you, then talk directly to him while he is neither occupied nor on the run. For some children, "whispering" into their ear may be more successful.

Also, many young listeners respond to all sensory stimuli—smell, sound, vision, touch. In other words, they are too attentive, but they are not selective. [Try it yourself. Consciously alert yourself to what you see, hear, feel, and touch simultaneously.] These children must be taught what we take for granted; that is, they must learn that by attending to only the key sounds, they will learn easier and more quickly. Therefore, reduce stimuli, except for what you want them to learn.

Further, processing time is different for many of these children. Failure to respond may be due to a delay between the actual request and the time the child can actually respond. Parents may demand a particular response, and if the child does not respond immediately, verbal embellishments are added to the initial command. This adds to the child's confusion. If he responds, but the response is not appropriate, it may be that the child "received" only part of the message—either the beginning or the end. Perhaps he was so absorbed in processing the first part that he "lost" subsequent information. Recognition of his failure to respond satisfactorily may cause the child to withdraw, to precipitate a frustration tantrum, or to make him feel inadequate as a person. So, learn to *wait* a reasonable length of time after giving a command.

Often when we have given a command or message, we have no notion of how much the child has understood. He may have confused the meaning of words so that the message made little sense to him. For example, the story is told of a child who, while crossing the street, was cautioned by his teacher to watch out for the wet tar. When he suddenly jumped back on the curb, he was questioned about this behavior and reported that he was warned to watch out for the white car. Therefore, when you give a command, observe the child's response closely—is it inappropriate, does he appear confused, is the execution vague? If the performance is · unsatisfactory, stop the child and ask (with a smile), "What did I tell you to do?" His answer may give you the information you need to know about the failure to perform properly, as well as to help him organize his thoughts and prepare for action.

The following recommendations are designed to help the child to listen, to retain, and to recall auditory information.

ACTIVITIES TO DEVELOP LEARNING TO LISTEN

A. *Learning to Listen*

1. Several times a day, play a game of being quiet and relaxed with eyes shut. The voice and the whole body should be quiet so that not a sound is made. Each child should be placed in the position where he is the most comfortable and relaxed; lying on the floor if necessary. At first, it may not be possible to maintain this silence for more than two seconds, but after a few weeks or months, it can be extended to two or three minutes.*

2. Once he can maintain reasonable quiet for 30 seconds or more, whisper a child's name and have him rise quietly and come to you. Continue until each child has a chance. At first it will be necessary to reintroduce the quiet relaxation after each child is called. As the child's listening ability improves, give him simple commands in the same whispered voice and position yourself in various areas of the room—sometimes near, sometimes far, sometimes in front of him, sometimes behind, etc.

3. To further encourage the child to listen and at the same time prevent yourself from falling into the habit of out-shouting him, make a habit of using a low, quiet tone of voice when presenting tasks or play items that the children really enjoy.

   Example: "Who would like to come help me?" "Who wants a balloon?" "Let's play ball," "Come see what I see," "Stand up now"

---

*Maria Montessori, *The Montessori Method* (New York: Schacken Books, 1964).

(after a prolonged period of sitting, etc.). Repeat once or twice or even whisper near a particular child's ear until he is aware of what you are doing.

4. Encourage listening by presenting interesting sounds:
    a. Whistle: Blow into the neck of a bottle partly filled with water.
    b. Thunder: Fill the bladder of a basketball or beach ball with pebbles and inflate. Shake it to get the proper rumble.
    c. Horses' hooves: Use one-half of a rubber ball and beat out the rhythm in box of dirt.
    d. Chimes: Tap with a stick on pipes, glass, clay pot, etc..
    e. Fire: Crackle cellophane.

B. *Learning to Listen and Locate*

1. Sound a noise-making target behind the child. Help him to learn to locate it by listening, then looking.

2. Have the child listen and decide the direction from which a more distant sound comes. Then have him look and find it. *Example:* Electric motor, refrigerator, running water, alarm clock, loud ticking clock, airplane, singing, cricket, ringing phone, typewriter, pencil sharpener, etc.

3. Blindfold the child and have him locate, then touch, an object as you sound it at various positions around, above, and below him. The sound should be distinct but not too loud or resounding, for the vibrations echo in all directions and cause confusion.

C. *Sound Discrimination*

1. Introduce two different sound-making targets. Let the child inspect and manipulate each.
    a. Sound one (under the table or any place out of the child's line of vision), then present both and have the child indicate which made the sound.
    b. Sound one from above or behind him.
    c. Introduce a new sound with one of the old familiar ones.
    d. Have him choose one out of three.
    e. Introduce more new sounds, one at a time.
    f. Ask for identification of the sounds with eyes closed.

2. Play games like "Simon Says" where the child must imitate your speech sounds, volume changes, rhythm alterations, etc.

3. Discrimination of voices: have the child identify the voices of members of the family or friends without visual clues. Begin with the person, later tape record the voices.

4. Volume discrimination: teach the child to distinguish which of two sounds is the louder.

   a. Use any instrument and have the child raise his hand or clap for the louder.

   b. Use voices, clapping, or sounds in the environment.

5. Games of word discrimination:

   a. Select simple pairs of common words where only a single sound element differs (coat-boat, king-ring, hat-hot, tea-key, etc.). Have available objects and pictures that match the words. Place objects or pictures on the table in front of the child, then ask for them by name. (This task presupposes that the child has already developed a vocabulary for all the words used.)

D. *Movement from Auditory and Visual Cues*

1. Imitating visual-auditory commands. The instructor gives the command, then performs, and the child imitates.

   a. Identification of body parts: "Put your hands on your head, . . . eyes, . . . feet," etc. (It is best to introduce one type of command such as "Put your hands on . . . ," but as soon as the children can understand and perform, use variations such as "Touch . . . ," etc..)

   b. Gross motor imitations: "stand, sit, kneel, crawl, walk, up and down, come, go, on, ŏff, in, out, open, shut," etc. Be sure to repeat the word at the moment the child performs so he relates the words to the activity; when an activity has an opposite, introduce only one until it is reasonably well learned, then the opposite. In fact, the child should be able to perform from verbal commands without visual cues before introducing the opposite. *Example:* The child should be able to perform the command "Put it on" in a variety of tasks before introducing "Take it off." Otherwise he is in danger of learning on and off without knowing the distinction between the two. Another example is the youngster who learned to use up and down verbally, but when she was performing a motor task of stooping and standing or raising and lowering an arm, she was as apt to say "up" when going down and "down" when coming up as she was to say it correctly. She had learned the two terms simultaneously and knew that they represented up and down movements, but she had not made the finer discrimination that each represented a different direction of movement.

E. *Auditory Clues*—activities in which clues are given to help the child identify visible, then hidden, goals

1. Association of objects or pictures of farm and domestic animals with the sounds they make. Don't complicate the activity by naming the animals. Just ask the child to choose the one that says "baa" or "bow-wow," etc. Try to make some sounds that are characteristically low, such as the cow's "moo," and some high, such as the cat's "meow." This furnishes an additional clue for discrimination.

2. Matching of familiar sounds, such as a clock or bell, with objects or pictures.

3. Have the child identify or choose by name one of a group of objects. The child is to identify by pointing or picking up. Use a group of pictures arranged on a table or in a book.
   a. Ask the child to point to or in some other way identify objects as you name them two at a time.
   b. Cover the pictures and ask for one (later two), then uncover and let the child choose. This will enhance memory.

4. Same as E.3, except that child identifies object or picture by its use.

5. Same as E.3, except that objects and pictures are identified by association. *Example:* "Give me the one I can eat with," "Give me the one you sleep in," etc.

6. Play "I Spy" or "Hide the Button." Tell the child he is to listen to you. When you make a sound loudly, he is near the hidden

goal, and when he is farther away, the sound will be softer and softer. Vary clues by saying:

a. "You're getting closer or farther away."
b. "You're getting hot or cold."

F. *Actions Performed from Auditory Clues Only*

1. Words:
   a. Perform a variety of activities from simple one and two word commands: "Come here," "No," "Sit down," "Go pottie," etc. The child may need to be helped through the activity at the moment it is spoken before he can see the relationship. *Example:* if he comes when you say "Come here," "Come to teacher," or "Come to mother," smile and let him know that he has responded appropriately. If, however, he shows confusion or runs the other way, have a second person guide the child to you as you smile, hold out your hands and say, "Come." This may need to be continued for several weeks or until the child relates the action to the word "come." Never, during this training period, require a child to come to you to be scolded or reprimanded, for thus you would discourage the action you wish him to learn.
   b. Simple sentences: give simple one sentence, one action commands. At this point introduce words denoting placement of self and objects in space. In-out, up-down, etc. Refer to D., *Movements from Auditory and Visual Clues,* pages 71–72.
   c. Increase number of words and commands. Remember that it may take 1 month to a year to move from a. to b., and b. to c. Use this time to elaborate and vary the task. That is, help the child learn many one word commands, for only then can you hope to integrate them into multiple commands.

2. Sounds:
   a. Use clues other than words for starting and stopping an activity. The activity may be a simple motor movement, a game, or a task. The task may be as simple as sitting still until a buzzer sounds.
   b. Introduce a sound for performing faster or slower, turning a corner, etc.
   c. Combine two or three of the above.

d. The child is to perform simple, predetermined rhythmic movements to the beat of a metronome or music with a good steady beat.

G. *Developing Auditory Memory*

1. Non-verbal response requiring memory through a short period of physical movement:

   a. Place three or four simple, familiar picture cards, propped up, on a tabletop or in the chalkboard tray. Seat yourself and the child about 4 feet away. Ask the child to get up and bring you a particular picture. When he can select each one correctly, substitute new pictures. Gradually add more pictures to the group.

   b. Increase the distance between the child and the pictures to 8 feet. Repeat the above.

   c. Increase the number of pictures you request at one time, starting with two pictures.

   d. Next remove the visual clues and have the child remember the command auditorally. Seat him about 8 feet from the cards and facing away from them. Repeat steps a., b., and c..

   e. Place the cards in an adjacent room and repeat steps a., b., and c..

   f. Increase the complexity further:

      (1) Give a sequence command, e.g. "Get the car and put it under the table."

      (2) Increase the time between your command and his execution of the task, e.g. "Jump, then get the car and put it on the chair."

2. Word and number sequencing:

   a. Have the child repeat unrelated words.

   b. Have the child repeat digits and/or letters after you. In order not to expect toő much of him, acceptable norms for auditory span are usually listed thusly:

Age	
3	3 digits
4	4 digits
5	5 digits
10	6 digits

Note: If it takes the child who is learning at a normal pace one year to move from 3 to 4 digits, do not expect the child with learning difficulties to move faster regardless of his age. (The child whose problem is that no one ever required memory tasks of him may progress quite a bit faster, but most children will not.)

No norms have been set for memory of 2 digits, but it is often wise to begin at this lower level.

   c. Increase the length of time between naming of the digits, words, or sounds, as the child demonstrates his competency, ¼ second to 2 seconds. (Learn to do without a timing mechanism; the mechanism is too distracting to the child.)

3. Read or tell a short, simple story containing two or more elements in a sequence, e.g. "Mother makes breakfast. John sets the table":

   a. Ask the child to retell the story. We are not interested in the refinements of sentence structure, but rather in the details presented and the sequential order.

   b. Ask the child "What did I say first . . . last?" Vary the order so that he knows he must listen to the entire story.

4. Sound sequencing:

   a. Select one syllable words (eyes, shoe, nose, etc.). Prolong the first sound, pause, then complete the rest of the word. Ask the child to point to, pantomime, or say the word that was just spoken. As the child becomes proficient, increase the length of the pause.

   b. Tell the child to say some nonsense syllable such as AN or AT just after you have pronounced another sound, e.g. you say "ppp" and the child says "AT." You ask what the word is that you have both made (PAT). Then go on to use other combinations, MAT, CAT, etc.

5. Carrying messages and accepting phone calls (these should be prearranged). If the child exhibits difficulty in "holding" a sequence of two, try either:

   a. Separating the two events emphatically by pausing between the instructions.

   b. Asking him to repeat the message to you before carrying it to another.

6. Jingles, nursery rhymes, songs, and stories. All children seem to enjoy the rhythmic sequencing of simple jingles, rhymes, songs, and stories:

   a. Encourage the child to repeat a sound or word that appears repeatedly in the material presented. *Example:* "ee-i-o" from "Old MacDonald."
   b. Encourage the repetition of final words in a line.
   c. Encourage the filling in of the final word in a line.
   d. Use one line songs, jingles, etc. and repeat them over and over until the child can repeat them alone. Invent your own and relate them to everyday activities.
      (1) "The snow is falling down."
      (2) "Pick up the toys, pick up the toys, now we pick up the toys."
      (3) "Round and round, round and round, Johnny's crayon goes round and round."
   e. Introduce simple two, then three line jingles or songs. Again relate them to everyday life.
      (1) "Garbage man, garbage man, pick up the garbage from the garbage can."
      (2) "Mister Mailman, Mister Mailman, do you have a letter for me, Mister Mailman—Please Mister Mailman, come and let me see."
   f. Read to the children.
      (1) Choose simple stories they can understand and relate to. The first ones should be one line to each picture.
      (2) Since the goal is to fasten the child's attention on the spoken word, choose stories containing noises or repeated sounds. If you cannot find ones adequate for the children's needs, make up your own.
      (3) Read slowly and distinctly.

REFERENCES

RECOMMENDED PHONOGRAPH RECORDS

Babbling Record, Bye Bye Baby Talk, Pacific Record Company, Children's Music Center, 2858 West Pico Boulevard, Los Angeles, California.

Babes in Toyland, Little Golden Records, 630 Fifth Avenue, New York, New York 10020.

Listening Activities, RCA Victor Records, 821 Broadway, New York, New York 10003.

Put Your Finger in the Air, J-4-187, Columbia Records, 545 Madison Avenue, New York, New York 10022.

Toy Symphony, RCA Victor Records, 821 Broadway, New York, New York 10003.

What's Its Name? Jean Utley, Interstate Printers, Danville, Illinois (record and workbook).

RECOMMENDED STORIES

Dr. Seuss Stories: *The Cat in the Hat,* New York: Random House, 1957.

The Cat in the Hat Comes Back, New York: Random House, 1957.

Dr. Seuss's ABC, New York: Beginner Books, 1963.

Hop on Pop, New York: Beginner Books, 1963.

One Fish, Two Fish, New York: Beginner Books, 1960.

P. D. Eastman: *Are You My Mother?* New York: Beginner Books, 1960.

Go, Dog. Go! New York: Beginner Books, 1961.

Robert Lopshire: *Put Me in the Zoo,* New York: Beginner Books, 1960.

Read to Me Storybook, Child Study Association of America, New York: Thomas Y. Crowell Company, 1947.

Rhymes for Children, Magnolia, Mass.: Expression Company.

Jack in the Box, Magnolia, Mass.: Expression Company.

The Three Bears

The Three Little Kittens

The Three Pigs

Monkey See, Monkey Do

Mother Goose

77

chapter 5

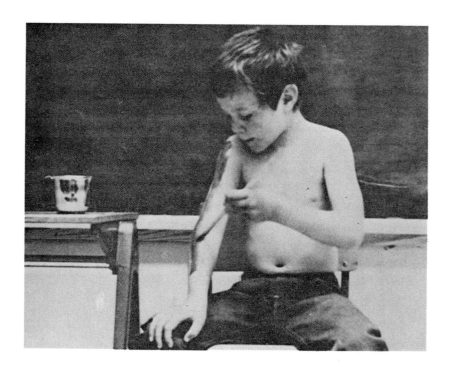

Tactual, visual, kinesthetic clues help to establish awareness of body parts.

Basic Adjustments

BALANCE AND POSTURE

The child begins to develop posture and balance immediately after birth as he uncoils from the intrauterine position. A little later he learns to control and balance his head, then the shoulders and midsection for seated balance, and finally he stands erect, maintains balance, and walks.

All the way the force of gravity is pulling at him and he constantly battles it as he pushes up to the standing position.

Equilibrium is the crux of the balance problem and it must be maintained in the many and varied positions that the child passes through as he learns balance. As a result, he develops a zero point, or a point of origin, out from which he can pivot and move and still maintain constant, flexible orientation to the earth's surface and the objects in his environment.

Without this gravitational axis, the child has no constant starting point from which to operate. This lack interferes with the development of awareness of self as well as with the stabilization of his environment, and learning becomes a slow, frustrating experience.

Adequate balance is also necessary to the child's safety; without it he can move neither quickly nor efficiently. Such a child is often tagged as being clumsy and is in danger of harm from external sources.

The following activities for development of balance and posture are listed sequentially. When not quite sure where to begin, the simplest approach is to start with No. I and have the child perform each item in sequence. Thus you can itemize those in which he needs special help.

ACTIVITIES TO DEVELOP BALANCE AND POSTURE

I. ON STOMACH

    A. *Head Differentiation*—have the child:

        1. Turn his face from mid position to one side, then to the other.

        2. Turn his face smoothly from side to side.

        3. Lift his chin off floor but not his chest.

        4. Lift chin and look about.

    B. *Trunk Awareness and Differentiation*—have the child:

        1. Lie perfectly still—begin with a few seconds, then extend to a minute or two.

        2. Roll to side, and then to back; each side.

        3. Lift his chest off the floor.

        4. Move whole body from side to side using:
           a. elbows and lower arm
           b. hands, arms extended

        5. Move just the upper trunk to differentiate the waistline. If necessary, hold the child at the hips to prevent movements of the entire body. Again, encourage pivoting with:
           a. elbows and upper arms
           b. hands

II. ON BACK

    A. *Head Differentiation*—encourage the child to:

        1. Turn face from side to side.

        2. Lift head and hold momentarily.

3. Lift head and look about.

4. Move head from side to side; face forward. Child's ear should aim for his shoulder.

B. *Trunk Awareness and Differentiation*—have the child:

1. Pivot upper trunk from side to side—*shoulders and hips should remain flat on floor.* Hold child's hips so only upper trunk moves. He should feel pull of muscles at waistline.
   a. As the child pivots to the side have him slide his hand down his side to touch his knee.
   b. Have him reach for an object on the floor to the far right or left. The object should be far enough away that real stretching takes place at the waistline.
   c. Have him just sway his upper trunk from side to side.

2. Lift his knees and point them first to the right, then to the left. Knees should move together but not as if they were locked together.

3. Reach across mid-area of body lifting only that shoulder; each side—use interesting objects to encourage reaching.

4. Pull self to sitting position—using instructor's hands, a pole, etc. The head should lift first, then the shoulders.

5. Do sit-ups, feet held down.

6. Reach his foot across mid-area of body lifting hip. (Shoulder remains in contact with floor or mat.) Here again, use interesting objects as a target for child to touch with his toes.

III. SITTING

A. *On Floor*

1. Sitting with legs crossed, child is to straighten back. Give as much help and cluing as necessary to make child aware of correct position. Then, have him draw his trunk erect—hold —release. Repeat, holding for longer periods of time.

2. Same as above with legs extended   in front. If muscles in back of legs are very tight, it n.a   ke months to work through this one.

3. Sit and sway from side to side (first w.th legs crossed, then with legs extended).

4. Sway fore and aft; both positions.

5. Encourage child to reach out in all directions while maintaining balance. Encourage movement at the waistline. Bending, stretching, and turning.

   a. Have him reach bilaterally—using both hands simultaneously.
   b. Have him reach unilaterally.

6. Gently push the child off balance in each direction. He is not to go limp and fall to the floor. Rather, encourage him to enervate muscles at waistline and in upper trunk to pull himself back to upright position. Hands should not be used.

7. Encourage child to sit perfectly still in each position.

8. Ask for head movements listed in activities to be performed on the floor, except that now the fore and aft movement can be more extensive.

9. Encourage child to scoot across floor by thrusting one leg forward, then the other.

B. *On Chair or Stool*—legs crossed, legs dangling

   1. Follow directions under III.A.—1 through 8. (Child is not to hold on to the chair for support.)

IV. ON KNEES

1. Same movements as in III.A.—1 through 7.

V. STANDING

A. *Procedure*

Place the child on a wooden block, stool, etc. that elevates him 4 to 6 inches off the floor. Surface should be narrow enough so that if the child steps, he wi be i. ,uired to step down to the floor, and narrow enough to discourage a wide stance.

1. Encourage the child to stand erect and still

2. Encourage him to manipulate parts of his body e maintains balance.

   a. Pat-a-Cake; move arms up and down.
   b. Reach out into all areas and grasp objects (. , . reach with arms and trunk): (1)bilaterally;(2)unil rally.
   c. Swing arms and upper trunk from side to side.
   d. Touch toes.
   e. Stoop and stand.
   f. Catch and throw ball; bounce and catch it.
   g. Stand on one foot; each foot.
      (1) Project elevated foot into variety of positions.
   h. Sway—right and left; fore and aft.
   i. Twist.
   j. Have the child place one foot on the block—stand erect and balance. Perform with each foot—use a variety of heights.
   k. Have child stand as in j., then lift foot from floor to block —up and down, sideways, forwards, backwards.
   l. Have child walk up and down steps. Discourage shifting from side to side with hips and swaying of body from side to side. The lead leg and hip should do all the work. Eventually, the child should be able to balance a beanbag, then a book, on his head.
   m. Variations: The following activities require a combination of coordinated movements and will therefore encourage the child to apply his newly learned movements.
      (1) Walking board with all its variations including items listed previously under Standing.
      (2) Balance board—variations as above.
      (3) Inclined plane—begin with 18 to 36 inch width.
         a. Standing still—facing up, down, right, left.
         b. Walking up and down, forward, backward, sideways.
         c. Perform as many as possible of the items under Sitting, Kneeling, and Standing.
      (4) Hiking over non-familiar terrain.

(5) Running, jumping, balancing on one foot, galloping, skipping, alternate jumping, etc..

(6) Many suggestions can be found in any elementary physical educational curriculum.

BALANCE BEAM EXERCISES*

1. Walk forward on beam, arms held sideward.

2. Walk backward on beam, arms held sideward.

3. With arms held sideward, walk to the middle, turn around and walk backward.

4. Walk forward to the middle of the beam, then turn and walk the remaining distance sideward left with weight on the balls of the feet.

5. Walk to center of beam, then turn and continue sideward right.

6. Walk forward with left foot always in front of right.

7. Walk forward with right foot always in front of left.

8. Walk backward with left foot always in front of right.

9. Walk backward with right foot always in front of left.

10. Walk forward with hands on hips.

11. Walk backward with hands on hips.

12. Walk forward and pick up a chalk eraser from the middle of the beam.

13. Walk forward to center, kneel on one knee, rise and continue to end of beam.

14. Walk forward with eraser balanced on top of the head.

15. Walk backward with eraser balanced on top of the head.

---

*BALANCE BEAM EXERCISES used by permission of Ray Page and the Physical Education Section of the Department of Curriculum Services, Office of the Illinois Superintendent of Public Instruction.

Note: Standard beam size: 2" x 4" x 10". Supports: 1" x 4" x 10".

As pupils improve in balancing skills, make another beam with the top tapered down to one inch in width; another with a half-inch top.

16. Place eraser at center of beam. Walk to center, place eraser on top of head, continue to end of beam.

17. Have partners hold a wand 12 inches above the center of the beam. Walk forward on beam and step over the wand.

18. Walk backward and step over wand.

19. Hold wand at height of 3 feet. Walk forward and pass under the bar.

20. Walk backward and pass under the bar.

21. Walk the beam backward with hands clasped behind the body.

22. Walk the beam forward, arms held sideward, palms down, with an eraser on the back of each hand.

23. Walk the beam forward, arms held sideward, palms down, with an eraser on the palm of each hand.

24. Walk the beam backward, arms held sideward, palms up, with an eraser on the back of each hand.

25. Walk the beam backward, arms held sideward, palms up, with an eraser on the palm of each hand.

26. Walk the beam sideward, right, weight on balls of feet.

27. Walk the beam sideward, left, weight on balls of feet.

28. Walk forward to middle of beam, kneel on one knee, straighten the right leg forward until heel is on the beam and knee is straight. Rise and walk to end of beam.

29. Walk forward to middle of beam, kneel on one knee, straighten the left leg forward until heel is on the beam and knee is straight. Rise and walk to end of beam.

30. Walk backward to middle of beam. Kneel on one knee, straighten right leg forward until heel is on the beam and knee is straight. Rise and walk to end of beam.

31. Walk backward to middle of beam, kneel on one knee, straighten left leg forward until heel is on the beam and knee is straight. Rise and walk to end of beam.

32. Hop on right foot, the full length of beam.

33. Hop on left foot, the full length of beam.

34. Hop on right foot, the full length of beam, then turn around and hop back.

35. Hop on left foot, the full length of beam, then turn around and hop back.

36. Walk to middle of beam, balance on one foot, turn around on this foot and walk backwards to end of beam.

37. Walk to middle of beam left sideward, turn around and walk to end of beam, right sideward.

38. With arms clasped about body in rear, walk the beam forward.

39. With arms clasped about body in rear, walk forward to the middle, turn around once, walk backward the remaining distance.

40. Place eraser at middle of beam, walk out on it, kneel on one knee, place eraser on top of head, rise, turn around and walk backward the remaining distance.

41. Walk the beam backward with an eraser balanced on the back of each hand.

42. Walk to middle of beam, do a right side support, rise and then walk to end.

43. Walk to middle of beam, do a left side support, rise and walk to end.

44. Place eraser on middle of beam. Walk out to it, kneel on one knee, pick up eraser and place it on the beam behind pupil, rise and continue to the end.

45. Walk to middle of beam, do a balance stand on one foot, arms held sideward with trunk and free leg held horizontally.

46. Place eraser at middle of beam, walk beam left sideward, pick up eraser, place it on right side of beam, turn around and walk right sideward to the end of beam.

47. Hold wand 15 inches above beam. Balance eraser on head, walk forward stepping over wand.

48. Hold wand 15 inches above beam. Balance eraser on head, walk backward stepping over wand.

49. Hold wand 15 inches above beam. Balance eraser on head, walk sideward right, stepping over wand.

50. Hold wand 15 inches above beam. Balance eraser on head, walk sideward left, stepping over wand.

51. Hold wand 3 feet high. Walk forward, hands on hips, and pass under the bar.

52. Hold wand 3 feet high. Walk backward, hands on hips, and pass under the bar.

53. Fold a piece of paper at the right angle so it will stand on the beam at the middle. Walk to paper, kneel, pick it up with teeth, rise and walk to end of beam.

54. Place paper as in 53., walk out to it, do a left side support, pick up paper with teeth and walk to end of beam.

55. Place paper as in 53., walk out to it, do a right side support, pick up paper with teeth and walk to end of beam.

56. Hop to middle of beam on left foot. Turn around on same foot and hop backward to the end of the beam.

57. Hop to middle of beam on right foot. Turn around on same foot and hop backward to the end of the beam.

58. Walk beam forward, eyes closed.

59. Walk beam sideward, eyes closed.

60. Walk beam backward, eyes closed.

61. Stand on beam, feet side by side, eyes closed and record number of seconds balance is maintained.

62. Stand on beam, one foot in advance of the other, eyes closed and record number of seconds balance is maintained.

63. Stand on right foot, eyes closed, and record number of seconds balance is maintained.

64. Stand on left foot, eyes closed, and record number of seconds balance is maintained.

65. Walk beam sideward left, eyes closed.

66. Partners start at opposite ends, walk to middle, pass each other and continue to end of beam.

67. Place hands on beam, have partner hold legs (as in wheelbarrow race) and walk to end of beam.

68. Same as 67., but partner walks with his feet on the beam, instead of the ground, straddling the beam.

69. "Cat Walk" on beam, walk on "all fours," hands and feet on beam.

ACTIVITIES TO DEVELOP BODY IMAGE
AND AWARENESS

To have body image is to know oneself, plus the ability to manipulate and control that self.

It is the child's knowledge of who and what he is; i.e. the parts and divisions of his body and their many possibilities for movement, synchrony of movement, and the relationship between oneself and objects in the environment. With this knowledge a child can do many things. Without it he will meet with frequent frustration, fear, tension, and failure.

The activities itemized here are specific to the development of awareness of self; however, nearly every activity listed in this book will add to and enhance it. As the child's awareness of himself is elaborated, his perceptions of the things about him will increase and integrated learning will become a greater possibility.

A. *Movement*

    1. Encourage the child to move about. (This need not be directed, but just movement for its own sake, involving any or all the parts of the body.)

    2. Movement of parts—head, arm, legs, trunk.

    3. Combination of parts—creep, crawl, wiggle, etc. over, under, through, between, behind, toward goals and through obstacles.

B. *Exploring Oneself*

    1. Encourage the child to look at and explore himself. Attract his attention to his own hands and feet, arms, legs, tummy, etc. To do this, it may be necessary to:

        a. Make sure that the child can see clearly at the necessary distances to explore his body.

    b. Stimulate the part—tap, squeeze, rub, etc..

    c. Add strong ocular stimuli—direct a light at the part, put a colorful patch or mark on the part, etc..

    d. Stress child's participation in bathing and dressing self. He is to look as he soaps an area or places a limb—use "Crazy Foam" or "soap crayons."

    e. Work before a mirror for variation.

    f. Stick small pieces of gummed paper on various body areas. Place one at a time and have the child locate and remove.

    g. Hide parts of his body and have him find them. *Example:* Cover with towel, sand, etc.

C. *Awareness of Movement in Other People*

    1. Encourage the child to watch you move. Here too, it may be necessary to use unusual means of attracting the child's attention. Try a., c., f., and g. above, applying the suggested ideas on the person to whom the child should attend.

    2. Experiment to see if the child will attend better when you are at a distance or close by.

D. *Imitation*

If, as the child observes your movements, he tries to imitate, well and good. Encourage him to carry through. If he seems frustrated and unable to reproduce the same movements in his body, help him move or have another person direct his movements. Let the child do as much as he can for himself. The directing hands should prevent wrong movements rather than direct the movement of the child. Have the child copy you as you:

    1. Move a body part or parts; pat-a-cake, wave, stick out your tongue, blow bubbles with the lips, make expressive facial movements, open and shut the mouth, move arm or leg up-down, etc. Later the child can imitate as you kick, stoop, sit, stand, shake your head, etc.

    2. Touch the parts of your body (name them as you do and encourage the child to touch any paired parts simultaneously, using both hands).

3. Rub parts of your body; the whole head, up and down an arm or leg, wash hands, etc.

4. Touch one body part to another; toe to mouth, toe to nose, head to knees, etc.

E. *Movements Upon Command*—ask the child to:

1. Look for, find, and touch body parts on himself, on others, on a doll, etc..

2. Move that arm or that leg—indicate by pointing (for the more advanced child, name right and left).

3. Move a part or parts into a given position. Refer to *Leg and Arm Differentiation,* pages 95–101.

4. Perform activities D. 1., 3., and 4. above.

5. Move and manipulate on command—reach, kick, swing arms, stoop, stand, sit, hop, jump, shake his head no-yes, blow, suck, chew, etc.

6. Identify a part by its use—what do you eat with, sit with, lick with, smell with, reach with, kick with, etc.

7. Relate a body part to objects in space—touch the table with your knee, etc.

8. Use a part or parts to propel an object through space—roll, throw, catch, or bounce the ball; pull the wagon; push the chair; catch the ball with both hands; push the ball with your elbow, head, knee, etc.; pick up the block, etc.

F. *Encourage Undressing and Dressing of Self.* Begin with items that permit visual contact as a body part enters the piece of clothing. First hold clothing for the child, then show him how to hold and perform. Encourage him to look. Begin in seated position.

G. *Projecting Body Image out from Self*—have the child:

1. Identify parts on another person, a doll, a teddy bear, etc.

2. Put a doll through many of the activities listed under Movement upon Command, E..

3. Dress and undress doll.

4. Assemble "people puzzles."

5. Play with sturdy "paper dolls."

6. Draw around another child on a large sheet of paper.

7. Draw around parts of self.

8. Add one or more features to a picture of a face.

9. Add all the features.

10. Add parts to a body (begin with trunk, head, arms and legs— later add feet, hands and joints). These may be made of wood, styrofoam, or heavy cardboard.

11. Make a man from a group of adequate parts. Use a variety of materials.

12. Identify from pictures, people (man, woman, boy, girl), parts, facial expressions, etc..

13. From memory, have the child add the missing parts to a figure of a man drawn on paper.

14. Ask the child to draw a man.

chapter 6

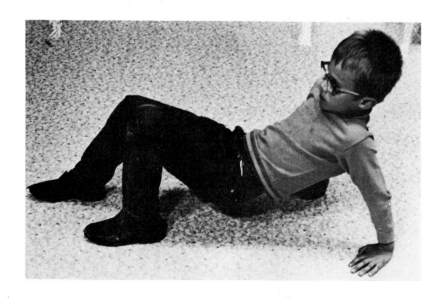

Experiments with different means of locomotion help the child to differentiate and coordinate body parts.

Differentiation and Locomotion

Differentiation is necessary to movement, and movement is essential to survival. The slow learner is one who, more often than not, has learned to move just adequately enough to survive in his immediate environment, but living for survival is no fun. It places the child under constant strain, building tensions and behaviorisms that further hamper learning.

As we work with all varieties of slow learners at the Achievement Center, the results indicate that, as a child learns to differentiate the parts of his body and elaborate and coordinate his movements, he does more than enhance his flexibility, posture, and poise. He also creates the possibility of increasing his perceptual abilities and his capability to make his intellectual capacity known. He improves his emotional stability and his social relationships.

The following activities are designed to help correct motor deficits. They are not all applicable to every child. It is necessary to analyze each child's deficits, then choose those pertinent to his problem.

By the same token, do not pick an isolated item or two and concentrate on them for weeks. Rather, organize a patterned approach and work out daily lesson plans. Help the child learn the basic movements pertinent to his problem, then introduce variations and encourage a great deal of experimentation to elaborate these and to coordinate them with the movements he already possesses.

Since differentiation means sorting out from, a differentiated part must be sorted out from the body mass, i.e. the part must be able to move without innervation in other parts of the body. Thus a child could perform many of the listed tasks and still not learn to differentiate, if he innervated and moved the trunk or other parts in order to move the specified limb. Such movement is global, the movement of the limb is not a specific movement sorted out from the whole; therefore the child's awareness of the movement of the specified limb is vague and confused because of the interference of the messages he is receiving from the other parts that are moving simultaneously. Once all the parts have been sorted out and the differentiated movements are habitual, the child will be able to move two or more parts in a coordinated fashion without one interfering with the other. When the coordinated movements become habitual, the child will be able to move through many and varied learning experiences and give his whole attention to the act of learning for he will no longer need to mentally control and direct his movements.

To get differentiated and coordinated movements, the child must learn to move out of relaxation. If, initially, the child cannot relax, that is move a part without tensing other areas of the body, the first task will be to help him do so, or at least to enable him to feel what it is to move a part without tension and/or overflow movement into other areas. At first this may require that someone hold in place all the parts of the body that are *not to be moved* as the child sorts out and moves the assigned part.

When working for differentiated movement out of relaxation, begin in the position in which the child is most comfortable; it may be lying on the floor or a mat, sitting cross-legged on the floor, or anchored in a chair.

In this section the activities are aimed at helping the child differentiate and coordinate his movements; first with the body stationary and then with it moving through space.

Leg Differentiation is listed first. It introduces one of the many groups listed under variations, that is, body positions.

In Arm Differentiation, where the number of possible movements are much greater, only the basic movements are listed with a list of activities that will help the child coordinate learned movements.

The section on Locomotion presents a series of differentiated, coordinated movements involving the movement of the whole body through space.

Following the above is a list of variations that can be applied to the activities in all three sections. These variations will help the child elaborate and integrate his movements and help the therapist avoid the pitfall of teaching "splinter skills." There are suggestions for:

1. Variations within the child.
2. Variations imposed upon the child.
3. Variations in the media, presentation, or environment.

It is necessary to keep in mind that what is a variation for an adult may be a whole new task for the child. When choosing variations, keep the child's needs, abilities, and difficulties in mind, for unless the task is presented in the child's present framework of learning abilities, it will be meaningless to him. He will avoid it, reject it, or respond emotionally to it, and little or no learning will result.

ACTIVITIES TO DEVELOP LEG DIFFERENTIATION

In the following activities the *body is not* to pivot or turn as the leg moves. The goal is to differentiate the hip area from the rest of the body.

A. *Hip Movement*—with bending of knee

1. On Back
   a. Draw knees up to chest, then extend or thrust out straight.
   b. Same as a. except that child is to make continuous circular thrusting movements.

2. On Stomach
   a. Draw both knees up under stomach and extend.
   b. Bend the knee and draw it up along side of body, on the floor, until it is in line with the hip, then extend.

B. *Hip Movement*—leg extended

For the child who has always initiated leg movement at the knee, it will be necessary to hold the knee in extension manually or with a simple splint until he becomes aware enough of the hip movement to initiate it properly himself.

1. On Back
    a. Lift the leg and lower it. $\circ\!\!\!\leftarrow\!\!\!\diagup$
    b. Move the leg out to the side along the floor, then return it to the mid-position beside the other leg.
    c. Swing the leg out to the side and back.
    d. Rotate the leg back and forth on the heel.
    e. Lift one leg and cross it over the other leg, touch floor if possible.
    f. Swing one leg over the other.
    g. Lift the leg and rotate it at the hip, making circles in the air with the foot.
    h. Place an object between the child's knees and tell him to hold it tightly.

2. On Stomach
    a. Perform items a. through h. above. In d. rotate the leg back and forth on the toes.

3. Lying on the Side
    a. Lift top leg and lower it.
    b. Place top foot in front of lower foot, slide the leg forward along the floor as far as possible, then back in place.
    c. Place top foot just behind lower foot and slide leg backwards.
    d. Lie with underneath leg bent at the knee, slide the upper leg fore and aft as far as possible.
    e. Lie with one leg on top of the other, lift the top one and:
        (1) Swing forward, then back to position.
        (2) Swing backward, then back to position.
        (3) Swing back and forth.
    f. Lift the top leg, rotate at hip, making circles in the air.

4. On Hands and Knees
    a. Extend a leg behind self, hold, return knee to floor.
    b. Extend leg, then move it:
        (1) Up and down.
        (2) From side to side.
        (3) In a circle.

5. On Knees
    a. Extend leg out to side and back.
    b. Lift one leg, and place foot flat on floor in front of self.
    c. Extend leg as far behind self as possible.

6. Standing—At first have the child stand where he can support himself against a wall, between door jambs, or at an exercise bar. When differentiation is adequate and balance permits, he can stand free to perform.

   a. Extend leg, knee straight:
     (1) Forward.
     (2) Backward.
     (3) Out to side.
   b. In (1), (2), and (3) above, extend and hold.
   c. Swing leg fore and aft.
   d. Lift one leg at hip joint, pulling heel off the floor.
   e. Slightly extend a leg forward, point the toe, and pivot the whole leg from the hip joint, making a semicircle with the heel, toe touching floor or leg extended out in front or to the side.
   f. Pivot a leg at the hip, making various sized circles.
   g. Place one foot on walking board as if to walk forward, lift body and weight on that leg, then lower and raise opposite leg at the hip joint. Have the child stand with opposite shoulder against the wall to steady him and avoid body sway until he can perform without support. Do not bend the knee of the leg that is standing on the board.

C. *Knee Movements*

1. On stomach—legs extended. Bend knees, draw foot up to buttocks, then extend slowly.

2. On back—legs extended. Keeping foot flat on the floor, slide it along the floor toward the buttocks, extend.

3. On side—With upper leg supported, child is to flex knee of lower leg, sliding foot along the floor toward the buttocks, then extend.

4. Standing—same movement.

D. *Ankle and Foot Movements*

1. In semi-reclining position, sitting on the floor or in a chair.

   a. Push toes away from the body—present something for the child to push against or reach for.
   b. Pull toes back toward self—present goal.

      c. Invert the foot so that the bottom of the foot is facing the opposite leg. Keep the leg straight so that inversion does not come from the knees. (Most helpful for child whose feet turn in.)

      d. Evert the foot so that the big toe side is down and the bottom of the foot faces out away from the body. (Ideal for feet that turn out.)

2. Standing or sitting in chair.

      a. Lift heels off floor (stand on tiptoes).

E. *Toe Movements*

1. Lying down, sitting, and standing.

      a. Place palm of hand, dowel, etc. under the ball of the child's foot (just under the toes) and ask the child to flex his toes down to it.

      b. Stabilize the foot and ask the child to extend or raise the toes.

      c. Have the child pick up small objects, folds of a towel, etc. with his toes.

ACTIVITIES TO DEVELOP ARM DIFFERENTIATION

A. *Shoulder Movements*

1. Move an arm in forward circular motion similar to the bilateral, symmetrical movement of the infant; elbows are bent and loose.

2. Move the hand up along the side of the body, extend it over head, then lower in same way.

3. Extend the arm to full extension out at side, then lower.

4. Extend the arm to full extension out in front, then lower.

5. Extend the arm to full extension down at the side of the body.

6. Extend the arm to full extension over the head, then down.

7. Move fully extended arm up and down in front of self.

      a. One quarter circle up and down.

      b. One half circle up and down.

8. Move fully extended arm up and down out to side of self.
   a. One quarter circle up and down.
   b. One half circle up and down.

9. Extend arm out to side at shoulder level, palms down, rotate the arm to bring palms up, reverse.

10. Extend the arm out in front, palms down, rotate the arm to bring palms up, reverse.

11. Extend arm out in front, move from center out to side and back again.

12. "Hunch" shoulders up and down.

13. Extend arm out in front, move it, in full extension, across front of the body until the hand extends out beyond the shoulder on the other side.

14. Lift hand to point out front, elbow bent, move arm fore and aft as child does to play "choo-choo".

15. Arm at side, swing it fore and aft.

16. Swing arm in circle in front of self.

17. Swing arm in full circle at side.

18. Extend arm out at side and swing in circles of various sizes.

19. Swing extended arm in circle over head.

20. Move just shoulder fore and aft.

21. Extend arm and rotate at shoulder.

22. Move shoulder in a circle.

23. Extend arm out in front—push and pull using only shoulder movement.

B. *Elbow Movements*

1. With arm extended in front of self, touch hand to shoulder, extend again—hold 2 or 3 seconds.

2. Arm extended out at side, bend elbow—touch hand to shoulder, extend again and hold.

3. Arm extended down at side—touch shoulder with hand, extend again.

C. *Wrist Differentiation*

1. With forearm stabilized on a board or table, child is to move the hand up and down freely, like a paint brush moving in vertical strokes over the edge of the table.

2. Move the hand freely from side to side.

3. Rotate the hand in a circular motion.
   a. To the right.
   b. To the left.

4. Move wrist as to screw and unscrew lids.
   a. To the right.
   b. To the left.

D. *Hand and Finger Movements*

1. Make a fist and open.

2. Spread fingers apart, then move them back together.

3. Bring tip of thumb and all fingers together.

4. Bring tip of thumb and pointer finger together.

5. Extend fingers and thumb to maximum and then relax.

6. Move thumb across the four fingers and back.

7. Touch each finger tip with tip of thumb—begin with pointer and move to little finger, then back.

8. Grasp a ball, then lift one finger at a time.

9. Close fist and release one finger at a time.

10. Extend hand, lower one finger at a time to form a fist.
11. Use a variety of grasping movements.
    a. Palmar.
    b. Thumb and four fingers.
    c. First finger and thumb.

E. *Activities to Coordinate Learned Arm and Hand Movements*

1. Shaking, rattling, pounding, pinching, picking, drumming, dropping an object, rolling an object, throwing, pushing an object, pulling, stacking, pouring, aligning, poking, squeezing, turning, cutting, kneading, winding, mixing, twisting, wringing, catching, bouncing, ball dribbling, reaching, petting, rubbing, placing, moving an object, picking up, releasing, finger plays.

ACTIVITIES TO DEVELOP LOCOMOTION

I. COORDINATION OF DIFFERENTIAL MOVEMENTS

A. *On the Stomach on the Floor:*

1. Wiggle like a snake, forward and backward.
2. Inch Worm—stretch upper trunk to move forward, then pull the lower trunk forward.
3. Push backwards with the hands.
4. Slide knees up under self and push body forwards.
5. Pivot on elbows.
6. Pivot on hands, arms extended.
7. Pull forward with elbows.
8. Pull forward, arms extended, hands flat on the floor.
9. Pull with arms and push with legs.
    a. Both arms and legs.
    b. Right arm and leg (moving in a circle).

    c. Left arm and leg (moving in a circle).

    d. Alternating.

10. Seal Crawl—Child is to use his hands to thrust chest off floor until elbows are straight, then propel self forward with the hands, dragging feet and legs.

B. *On the Back:*

    1. Push with feet and pull with arms.

    2. Push with arms and pull with feet.

    3. Use just arms or legs.

C. *Rolling:*

    1. Roll from back to side and hold.

    2. Roll from back to stomach and hold.

    3. Roll from stomach to side and hold.

    4. Roll from stomach to back and hold.

    5. Roll over and over.

        a. Lead with head.

        b. Lead with arm.

        c. Lead with leg.

D. *Sitting:*

    1. Scoot forward, backward, sideways, or in a circle.

        a. Use hands and feet.

        b. Use just hands.

        c. Use just feet.

    2. Move forward and backward using alternating leg thrusts.

    3. Scoot up and down stairs.

        a. Using leg thrust.

        b. Using arm thrust.

        c. Using both.

E. *Hands and Knees:*

1. Move across the floor on hands and knees in as many directions as possible.
   a. Using unilateral movements, right arm and leg, then left arm and leg.
   b. Cross-lateral—right arm, left leg; then left arm, right leg.
   c. Propel self forward with legs alternating as hands push bilaterally on a large block.
   d. "Three-legged."
      (1) With one hand, push a wheeled toy, block, etc. about the floor while using the other three limbs for locomotion.
      (2) Use both legs and one arm, holding the other arm off the floor.
      (3) Use two arms and one leg, lifting the other leg like a wounded dog. It may be necessary for a second person to hold up the unused leg.

F. *Hands and Feet:*

1. Bear Walk—all directions.

G. *Knees:*

1. Walk on knees, body erect; forward, backward, and sideways. Do not permit the child to rotate the body or move at an angle.

H. *On Feet:*

1. Walk.

2. Run.

3. Hop.

4. Jump.
   a. Vary as many ways as possible.

VARIATIONS OF ACTIVITIES

A. *Vary the Parts to be Moved*—have the child perform using:

1. Two limbs simultaneously:
   a. Bilateral—arms or legs.
   b. Unilateral—arm and leg on a side.
   c. Cross-lateral—left arm, right leg.

2. Each part individually—head, arm, leg, elbow, wrist, hip, shoulder, hand, fingers.

3. Upper and lower trunk—separating the trunk at the waistline.

B. *Vary the Positions of the Body:*

1. Lying down on back, stomach, each side.

2. Sitting:
   a. On floor—legs straight, legs open, Indian fashion, on feet, etc.
   b. On variety of objects—blocks, stool, balance board, chair, etc.
   c. In things—boxes, water, etc.

3. Hands and knees—on floor, on objects, in things.

4. Kneeling—on floor, on objects, in things.

5. Standing—on floor, on objects, in things.

6. Hanging—with arms, legs, arms and legs, suspended at the waistline.

C. *Vary the Movements*—have the child move his body, a part or parts:

1. Up, down, in, out, over, under, back and forth, towards goals or through obstacles.

2. To swing, sway, push, pull, shake, turn, etc.

3. To reach, point, touch.

4. To grasp or release.

5. To push, pull, or thrust.

6. In imitation of objects, animals, etc.—sway like tree, fly like bird, walk like animal.

D. *Alter the Extremities:*

1. Weighting—to distort gravity.
   a. Symmetrical—both hands, both feet, across shoulders or head.
   b. Asymmetrical—one arm, one leg, arm and leg on one side, òr weights both sides simultaneously with more weight on one side than on the other.

2. Increase or decrease numbers: one leg, two legs and one arm, both hands and feet, etc.

3. Alter relationships:
   a. Vary the position of limbs (i.e., ask for the same movement with the arm down, extended to side, extended out front, etc.).
   b. Alter position of the trunk—tilt forward, backward, etc.

4. Increase bulk—finger and hand puppets, appendage wrapped in burlap, swim fins, skate boards, etc.

5. Increase length—have the child perform with an object that extends the reach of his arm or leg.
   a. With stick or pole—reach out to point to or follow a target.
   b. Use broom, mop, or sweeper—to follow lines, point to targets, clean up sand, bits of paper, etc.
   c. Walk on stilts.

6. Leverage changes—pedal cars, walkers, tricycle, toy handcars, Irish mail, roller skates, jumping shoes, pogo sticks, crepe soles, one foot in a small box, etc.

E. *Alter the Force of the Movements*—smooth and easy, thrusting hard, pushing against pressure, etc.

F. *Alter the pace of the Movements:*

1. Slow, fast.

2. Let the child set his own rhythm.

3. Have him perform to a variety of external rhythms, counting, clapping, metronome, music.

4. Use the trampoline.

5. Keeping in a performing line.

6. Taking turns.

G. *Vary the Presentation:*

1. Move the child who cannot move himself.

2. Hold out extraneous or overflow movement.

3. Have the child imitate.

4. Vary the commands:
   a. Auditory, visual, and tactual.
   b. Any two of the above.
   c. Any one of the above.

5. Present goals for the child to move toward and for the child to follow.

H. *Vary the Environment:*

1. Large and small spaces.

2. In isolation, amid distractions—first slight, then normal.

3. Alone—with others (one, two, or more).

4. Classroom, home, pool, playground, etc.

I. *Vary the Media:*

1. Terrain—stairs, stepping stones, hills, ladders, trees to climb, etc.

2. Submersion in a media:
   a. buoyancy—pool or tank of water.
   b. suction—mud, soft clay, papier maché, deep snow or sand, etc.

3. Surface changes:

   a. Alter surface friction—on concrete, in grass, in snow, in sand, on wet surfaces.

   b. Interrupt gravity temporarily—trampoline, jumping board, spring and mattress.

   c. Limit the surface—walking boards and inclined planes of various widths, lengths, and heights. Walk a line, etc.

   d. Shift the surface—balancing boards, T-boards, swinging bridges, rope-climbers and ladders, rubber tires, large inner tubes, etc.

   e. Introduce obstacles that require the child to wiggle, squirm, crawl, creep, climb through, under, over, around, between, up, down, in, out, etc.

SWIMMING POOL ACTIVITIES*

The pool is an excellent medium of variation for the presentation of many activities performed by the child in other areas. However, it also offers an opportunity to perform movements that cannot be practiced elsewhere. The bouyancy of the water greatly reduces the force of gravity and prevents the child from injuring himself. In addition, the water offers resistance to movement, thus increasing the tactual-kinesthetic information coming from movement of the limbs.

Listed here are only a few of the many possibilities:

1. Pouring of water

   a. While the child sits on the side of the pool, pour water over various parts of his body, and have him name the part.

   b. Have the child pour the water as you name the part.

2. Help the child learn to get *himself* into and out of the pool one way or another.

3. Movement in the water

   a. While sitting along the edge of the pool, have the child place different parts of his body in the water and move them about.

   b. While supported on back or stomach, sitting, kneeling, or standing in the water, have the child move the various parts of his body. (Check differentiation of arms and legs for ideas.)

Teaching Aids: life belts, balls, hula hoops, ropes, weighted objects, rafts, water toys.

4. Movement through the water

   a. Have the child perform a variety of locomotion patterns.
   b. Have the child propel a variety of objects through the water.
   c. Hand-walk along the side of the pool, right to left, left to right, sliding hands, lifting hands, crossing one hand over the other.
   d. Hold onto the ledge and walk the feet up until the toes are out of the water, then back down again.

   Games: Ball play of all kinds, Tag, "Here We Go Round the Mulberry Bush," "Tug 'o War," Relay Racing, "Hokey Pokey," etc.

5. Submersion of the face—have the child:

   a. Bob his face in and out of the water.
   b. Blow bubbles on surface of water.
   c. Relax knees and submerge whole body until head is covered.
   d. Blow bubbles under the water.
   e. Work on rhythmic breathing as the face goes in and out of the water.

   Games: "Jack in the Box," Stoop Tag, Dodge Ball, etc.

6. Use obstacles set up in the pool for the child to step over, duck under, weave in and out and around, push, pull, etc.

TRAMPOLINE ACTIVITIES

The trampoline offers multiple possibilities for variation in helping the child further his development in balance, body image, differentiation of body parts, coordination, and spatial orientation.

The device itself, in the give of the canvas, demands variations in balance. Body image and differentiation are enhanced each time a part or parts of the body come in contact with the canvas. Quite often these are parts of the body that have never before come in contact with a reasonably solid surface in just that way. Coordination is required if the child is to maintain the various positions on the canvas.

Most children have some sort of internal rhythm but have difficulty adjusting to or imitating an external rhythm. On the trampoline the rhythm is dictated in part by the device itself and the child must, in order to perform, adjust his responses to the pattern set by the device. The child's orientation is elaborated as the device tosses his body about in space.

The trampoline also supplies a new terrain on which the child is more likely to incorporate newly learned movements. For instance, the child has been walking, running, jumping, etc. on floors, sidewalks, and earth all his life. He has learned set patterns of movement, many of them inadequate. After an intensive training program he learns to move more adequately during the training but does not transfer the newly learned movements to familiar tasks because the old patterns of movement are habitual. However, if he is put on the trampoline and asked to move, he cannot move in the old way; he has to elicit different movement patterns and the newly learned ones are called into action. After a while they become so extensive to him that he transfers them via common elements to the old familiar tasks.

When trampoline activities are first introduced, encourage, in fact, insist that the child get onto the device himself. If someone puts him upon it, his orientation is disturbed and he becomes lost in space, unsure of the gap between him and the floor. Do not be apprehensive of the very young child or the child who is performing at an early level; be patient and he will find his way up and be happier with his success than he would have been with your help.

Once the child is on the canvas have him:

First Step: Maintain balance in one place. Child should experiment on all fours, kneeling with back straight, standing erect.

Second Step: Make him, using the same positions as above, shift his weight from side to side and fore and aft.

Third Step: He can move about the canvas, again in each of the previous positions. Have him explore the width and length of the canvas plus the give of the canvas as one, then another, limb leaves the surface while moving about.

The child may spend weeks experimenting with these exploratory movements and learning about the device.

Fourth Step: Have the child learn to control the body and its parts, maintaining his balance and orientation as someone else moves the canvas up and down.

(This can be done with a person on each side of the trampoline bouncing the canvas or one person up on the trampoline lightly jumping as he moves about the child on the canvas.) The child can be on his back, stomach, sitting with legs out straight and hands flat on the canvas, on hands and knees, kneeling or standing.

Bouncing is the most important activity of the trampoline and from this point the child should begin bouncing himself. If executed with balance and rhythm, the
child will utilize 90% of the value of the device.

a. The symmetrical-bilateral child automatically alter-
   nates if he does nothing but shift or move about on
   the canvas and advances even further as he does
   alternate jumping.

b. The asymmetrical child must break out of his asym-
   metry as he jumps bilaterally if he is going to maintain balance.

c. Differentiation and coordination of the 4 quadrants
   is introduced as the child moves about on all fours,
   but this is perfected as he uses the arms in a variety
   of patterns as he bounces.

Fifth Step: Bilateral Bouncing and Jumping

a. Feet do not leave canvas.

b. Feet leaving canvas.

c. Starting and stopping on command. (Teach the child
   to stop by bending his knees to take out the spring).

d. Catching and throwing ball, bean bag, etc. while
   bouncing or jumping.

e. Incorporate arm movements in the activity.
   1. Clapping—in front of body, behind, from front
      to back, between legs, etc. in rhythm with jump.
   2. Moving arms up and down at side, and in front in
      rhythm with the jump.
   3. Swinging arms at sides, forward and backward
      and across front of body and back.
   4. Swing arms in full circles—at sides forward and
      backward; in front of self in overlapping circles.
   5. Place hands on shoulders, then move hands out
      and back in various directions—again keeping
      time with the jumping.

(a) Out to side and back.

(b) Out to front and back.

(c) Over head and back.

6. Jump feet apart and together.

7. Perform jumping jacks, varying the arm positions as in b., c., and e.

Sixth Step: Alternate and Unilateral Jumping

a. "Mexican Hat Dance" movement—legs alternating front and back.

b. Alternate Jumping

1. From one foot to the other.
   (a) One jump on each foot.
   (b) Two jumps on each foot.
   (c) Two on one foot and one on the other—reverse.

2. On one foot for extended periods of time (30-60 seconds).

3. Setting and changing the jumping pattern from visual clues. Instructor holds up fingers indicating the number of jumps to be performed on each foot—2—2, 1—1, 2—1, 1—2, etc.

As soon as the child begins to perform on his feet, it is necessary to have two, and when possible, four spotters about the trampoline to prevent any possibility of danger. However, the possibilities of a child being hurt are minimal if a few sensible precautions are taken.

chapter 7

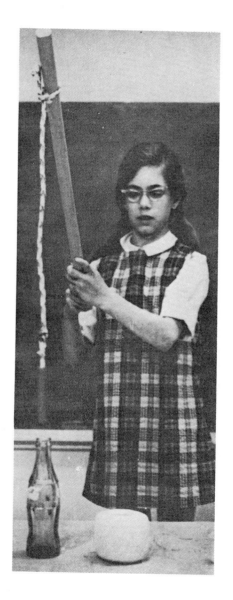

The visual-motor match must be general-ized when the length of the arm is artifici-ally increased.

Ocular Motor Coordination

The infant learns to use his eyes and hands as a unit at a very early age. He spends hours, weeks, even years watching his hands perform as they explore textures, edges, surfaces, in fact, all the facets and dimensions of his world. This information becomes very important for future academic learning. If the child does not learn to use his eyes and hands in unison, learning often suffers. The following activities suggest possible means of helping the child develop his visual motor controls.

Because most of the children who have ocular motor problems also have gross motor problems, including inadequate or rigid balance, it is best to begin all eye-hand activities with the child lying on his back on the floor. This permits the child to differentiate eyes, hands, and arms without concentrating on balance control. Some children, however, are more secure in the sitting position. If so, work should begin there. Be sure the child is well anchored in the chair so he can again concentrate on the task rather than on balancing and maintaining his position on the chair. Most children submit readily to being strapped into a chair if it is first explained that no punishment is involved. You are only helping him relax so he can better attend to the task. Calling it a "seat belt" makes it even more acceptable.

ACTIVITIES FOR OCULAR MOTOR COORDINATION

A. *Fixations**

1. Therapist holds a target in each hand 12 to 18 inches in front of the child. One should be at the midline and the other 6 to 12 inches out in the periphery.

   a. Vary the targets and method of contact.
      (1) Use two squeaky toys and encourage the child to reach out and squeeze one, then the other.
      (2) Use two tap-bells and have the child reach out and tap one, then the other.
      (3) Use other sound making targets. Sound one, have the child reach out and touch it, then sound the other and have the child touch it. He is to keep his eyes on one target until the other is sounded.

   b. Vary the distance. Have the child sit on one side of the room and fixate and point from target to target on the other side of the room (look at the chair, then at the television).

   c. In the above activities, have the child:
      (1) Use his right hand when fixating from the midline out to the right and the left hand to the left.
      Work for a period of time in each area, not back and forth across the midline.
      (2) Change the outer target so that the child can practice vertical, lateral, and diagonal movements.
      (3) Perform both monocularly and binocularly. Note: When performing monocularly, begin by having the child use the right eye with the right hand and the left eye with the left hand. Later for variation, have him use right hand, left eye, and reverse. Always end this session with both eyes and hands involved as in 2.-a. and b. below.
      The monocular training is introduced only long enough and often enough to make the child aware of the performance of each eye.
      (4) Permit the child to move his head as he looks from one target to another until he understands what is required

---

*Fixation, pursuit, and convergence defined in Glossary.

and is comfortable in the task. Then hold his head to encourage eye movements.

2. Hold the targets so that the child's eyes must cross the midline each time he moves his eyes from one target to the other. Begin with a very short distance between targets and gradually extend. With both eyes involved, the child is to:

    a. Touch the right target with the right hand and the left target with the left hand. Continue this activity until he can do it rather easily and the eye movements across the midline are reasonably smooth.

    b. Clasp his hands together and use the extended "pointer" fingers to touch each target.

    c. Use just the right or left hand and both eyes.

    d. In a., b., and c. above:

        (1) Move the targets so the child can practice vertical and lateral movements. Diagonal movements can be introduced after vertical and lateral movements are reasonably smooth.

        (2) Repeat in each direction several times.

        (3) In each step, encourage the child to hold visual contact with the target for several seconds before moving to the next target.

        (4) Have the child fixate along a series of targets pointing to each. *Example:* Line up in sequence a ball, block, ball, block, etc. and have the child fixate on and touch each one as you or he names it.

3. Hold a large ball, or any other object which is attractive to the child and large enough to require the use of both hands, in your hand and within easy arm's reach of the child. Encourage him to look at it as he reaches out to grasp it with both hands, then to look at your hands as he gives it back.

    a. Present the ball directly in front of the child and below eye level.

    b. Present it from any point within an area no wider than the child's shoulders so that he must reach across his midline with the one hand when grasping with both hands.

Since actual visual-motor training can be done only during a small portion of the child's day, it is necessary to encourage him to explore, play, and work using his eyes and hands, simultaneously, in many tasks.

Activities that encourage the child to fixate his eyes on his hands as he works are many and varied. A few are listed here:

1. Exploration of self as in B.1.a.—g. in *Activities to Help Develop Body Image and Awareness,* pages 88–89.

2. Exploration of a variety of objects.

3. Looking and pointing at pictures, randomly or from one to another in a row of pictures or objects.

4. Pointing out various objects in the room as they are named.

5. Playing with form boards, simple puzzles, and pegboards.

6. Bead stringing.

7. Placing of knives, forks, and spoons in separate trays.

8. Poking at soap bubbles in the air.

9. Putting plastic forms on dowels. ⊚ ▭ △ ══

10. Sorting and aligning many objects.

Most of the above activities can be adapted for specific training when needed. The pegboard is a good example. Place the pegboard directly in front of the child, then present him with a peg and tell him to take it. If he locates the peg with his eyes, then looks away as he reaches out to grasp it, quickly moving the peg a short distance. Continue to move it each time he looks away until he looks and grasps simultaneously. Then tell him to place it in the board. Once the child can perform this simple task, you can introduce variations:

1. Set two pegs as goals and ask the child to place the pegs in the intervening holes as you present pegs to him one at a time. Set the goals for vertical and horizontal lines.

2. As the child progresses and shows evidence that he is ready for more advanced tasks, set the goals for a variety of patterns:
   a. Joining lines. ⊢ ∟ ⌐ ⊤
   b. Intersecting lines. ⊥ + —+
   c. Diagonal, joining, and intersecting lines. / V X Z △

B. *Pursuits*

1. Target
   a. Hold a target about 20 inches before the child's eyes. Ask him to watch it wherever it goes.
   b. Choose a target to fit the child's needs. The addition of auditory clues may be necessary.
   c. Have the child follow the target with one hand, then the other, and with both hands interlocked with the pointer fingers extended to follow the target.

2. Movements
   a. Move the target several times in each of the following directions:
      (1) Laterally.
      (2) Vertically.
      (3) Diagonally.
      (4) In a circle.
   b. The extent of the eye movements will vary. Find the length of movement at which the child performs best in each direction. Begin work here and extend to a maximum of 20 to 30 inches.
   c. Move the target in an arc, keeping it 18 to 24 inches in front of the child's eyes at all times, for directions (1), (2), (3) in 2.a. above, thus keeping the eye-target distance constant.
   d. Keep the child in the center of the task.
   e. If the child moves his head, ask him to hold it still. If he cannot, hold it for him.
   f. Watch the eyes carefully to determine whether both eyes are pointed directly at the target. If the child loses the target, immediately stop the target and ask the child to refixate on it.
   g. If the child has difficulty pursuing across the midline or if there is a jerk or hesitation as the eyes cross, use the following sequences:
      (1) Variety of movements from the midline out to the left, then to the right, each hand involved.
      (2) Very short movements across the midline, both hands involved.
      (3) Gradually extend length of movements.
      (4) Use only one hand.

3. Position

   a. Begin the activities with child on his back or on the floor or comfortably anchored in a chair.

4. Fatigue

   a. Because these activities make complex neuromuscular demands upon the child, he may easily become fatigued. Therefore, the training activities should be practiced for only short periods (3-5 minutes) of time but can be practiced several times a day.

5. Activities that encourage visual pursuit of motor movements.

   a. Chalkboard

     (1) *Scribbling*—Offer the child many opportunities to scribble. Encourage smooth, free flowing arm movements that involve elbows and shoulders rather than just the hand and wrist. Have the child use each hand, then both hands simultaneously. If the child rejects the chalk or cannot maintain a grasp on it, cover the board with chalk and have him use the palm of his hand to make designs in the chalk dust, or let him use the very large round chalk or blocks of chalk that he can grasp in his palm. Occasionally ask the child to step back and observe that which he has scribbled and to follow portions of it with his finger. In the normal child, the art of scribbling advances through several stages before the child is ready to reproduce forms. The progression from the first try at the board to the creation of form takes 2 to 3 years.*

     (2) *Drawing*—Have the child draw lines between goals, vertical and lateral. Stress continuity and the production of single lines with attention to starting and stopping on the goals. Have him draw from right to left several times, then from left to right. Have him use each hand and make sure that he remains in the center of the task and moves from target to target with eyes and hand without moving his head or body. Since, at this point, we are interested in ocular motor training, it may be necessary to seat the child at the board if other motor problems are interfering—inadequate balance, for example. (For best results, the board should be slanted forward slightly and

*R. Kellogg, *What Children Scribble and Why* (Palo Alto, Calif.: N. P. Publications, 1955).

high enough that the child's knees fit under the board.)
Use a variety of ways to entice the child to draw.

(a) From dot to dot. •———————•

(b) Between matching objects.

(c) To associate object to action.
     Example: Have the boy get the ball.

(d) Use the Dot Game.*
(e) Single continuous circles:
     1. In both directions.
     2. With each hand.
     3. Vary the size.
     4. Vary the speed.
     5. Encourage the child to keep his eye on the trace.
(f) Double continuous circles:
     1. In, out, parallel in both directions.

     2. Encourage synchrony of movement between the
          two hands.
     3. Circles should not touch in the center.
     4. Encourage the child to keep his eyes in the cen-
          ter, monitoring both circles simultaneously.

(3) *Tracing***—Have the child trace over a motif that is
     placed directly in front of him. It can be traced with
     either hand and in both directions. Vary the size of the
     motif and the speed of tracing. At first, make the outline
     quite wide and gradually decrease to a chalk trace.

(a) Lines, straight, curved, angled.   ———   ⌒⌒

(b) Repeated letters.

(c) Nonsense motifs.

(d) Forms.   ○ □ △ ▢ ◇

(e) Combinations of letters.

(f) Words—go from simple to complex.

---

*Newell C. Kephart, *The Slow Learner in the Classroom* (Columbus, Ohio:
Charles E. Merrill Publishing Company, 1960), p. 169f.
**Supplementary reading: *Ibid.,* pp. 146-150 and 241-258.

b. Pegboard
   (1) Instead of having the child fill in between goals on pegboards as outlined under A. *Fixations,* present the design drawn on a sheet of paper. Have him trace it with his finger several times, then reproduce it on the pegboard.
   (2) Next have him copy his design on paper or chalkboard. Compare to original copy at each step.

c. Variations:
   (1) Vary the chalkboard drawing and tracing, and the pegboard activities by having the child:
      (a) Creep and walk around motifs, letters, and words drawn on large, long sheets of paper placed on the floor.
      (b) As he creeps or walks have him push an object (block, pole, etc.) along the motif.
      (c) Have the child arrange the designs on the floor with a rope or lengths of board.
      (d) Have the child reproduce the designs at the table, with his finger or hand in clay or finger paints, with ropes of clay, with blocks, tongue depressors, etc.

C. *Convergence*

1. Hold a small target (an item that will readily attract the child's attention) directly in front of the child's eyes at a distance of 18 inches. Ask the child to look at the target as you move it in to about 4 inches from his nose.

2. The child may have difficulty converging, that is fixing both eyes on the moving target and holding them there. If so:
   a. Move the target in just short of the point where one or both eyes lose the target, then out again.
   b. Gradually work in closer.
   c. Have the child glance from a near target to one 10 to 15 feet away. Begin with the second target directly in front of him. Later, diagonal movements can be introduced.
      (1) The child should be able to release his eyes from each target easily and smoothly and should move the eyes directly to the other target and fixate without any extraneous movements.
      (2) Note: There are some children who cannot converge or obtain fusion at 18 inches. For such a child the target is presented at a greater distance.

chapter 8

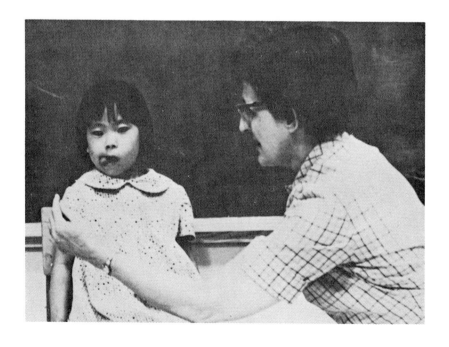

Control of the tongue, lips, and jaws is important for speech.

Speech Readiness*

By Sylvia B. Kottler

To master the art of speaking, the young child must first learn:

1. How to move and manipulate the musculature of the mouth, jaw, lip, and tongue.

2. He spends hours, weeks, and months practicing these movements.

3. He learns to name objects, then actions, and eventually sentences as his structured world gives him something to talk about.

The child with learning difficulties is often slow to speak or his speech is not articulate because, due to an overall inadequacy of the motor system, he has difficulty learning to swallow, suck, chew, and manipulate the tongue. He often does not get around to using sounds because he needs to concentrate so completely on the gross motor movements necessary for getting about in his environment that there is no time to concentrate on speech. Quite often, according to the report of parents, such a child develops speech and language according to the norms until he begins to walk. It is not unusual for a child to let up on speech as he concentrates on the art of walking. Since the child with motor problems often spends months (maybe years) concentrating on the art of walking,

---

*This chapter is adapted from two papers, "Speech Readiness I" and "Speech Readiness II," prepared by Sylvia Kottler, Speech Pathologist, Achievement Center for Children, Purdue University.

he never gets back to the business of speaking. If he does, the demands made of him are too far advanced and he cannot master the gap between that which he had learned and that which is now being required of him. As a result, he does not speak or his speech is inarticulate and inadequate.

Therefore, when helping the slow learner with speech problems, it is frequently necessary to start at the beginning with the sucking, swallowing, chewing movements and tongue manipulation so necessary for eating and articulate speech.

The function of speech can be developed and trained only if the oral musculature becomes proficient on the vegetation level first. Observe how the child handles his food; does he chew on one or both sides; does he wipe it off with his fingers; can he sip through a straw; how does the tongue thrust the food toward the throat for swallowing; does he eat a variety of foods necessary for good nutrition as well as for exercising the oral muscles? For any child who requires more experience in oral motor manipulations, the following activities are suggested:

ACTIVITIES FOR ORAL MOTOR MANIPULATION

I. SUCKING

A. *Tactile Stimuli*

1. Touch first the lips, then above and below the lips, and last, the cheeks.

B. *Puckering*

1. Gently place fingers around the lips and spread the lips apart. (This provokes a contrary movement—a pucker.)

C. *Straw Sucking*—Material: very cold fluids of interesting tastes and good odor.

1. If a plastic straw is inadequate because the child bites down on it, or if his lips cannot obtain sufficient closure to surround it tightly, procure a piece of rubber tubing (3/8 inch in diameter) from a surgical supply store.

2. If the lips are too weak for 1. here, start with straws sealed with wax into a large spool or rubber stopper. As the lips become more efficient, introduce smaller spools until the child uses the straw alone.

D. *Teaching How to Suck*

1. Place a small piece of plastic straw into a liquid. Put your finger over the hole, thus holding in the liquid, lift liquid-filled straw and place it into the child's mouth. (This is merely associating a good taste with the straw.) Next, lower the end of the straw a little below the horizontal so the liquid will not be free flowing, but it can be sucked in easily. Give the child visual and auditory clues of hearty smacking and suction noise of the tongue. Let him know you are pleased with his effort. Repeat often and very gradually alter the direction of the straw until it is in a vertical position.

2. Suck thick liquids such as soup or milk shakes through a paper straw routinely.

3. Practice sucking from a different container—pop bottles, glasses, cups, bowls, etc.

4. Do not *introduce* straw sucking at meal time, but preferably when the child is relaxed and you are unhurried.

II. BLOWING

A. *How Child Blows*

1. Observe the child to determine how he blows; is it a snort, a huff, an F-position expulsion, or the preferred "P"? The following are listed in order of difficulty: birthday candles, cotton balls or tissue paper on a mirror, bubbles, whistles, toy horns, birthday poppers, harmonica, Ping-Pong balls, pinwheels, musical instrument, balloons.

III. CHEWING—involves the coordination of the muscles, bones, and joints of the jaw, lips, and tongue.

   A. *The Jaw*—in normal chewing, the jaw makes rotational and grinding (side to side, forward and backward) movements and opening and closing of the mouth.

      1. Biting strength—bite off food (carrots, raw potatoes, etc.) with front teeth rather than with molars.

      2. Chew food on each side equally. At first, it may be necessary to reinforce the chewing with auditory clues. Thus, you will say, "Chew—chew, chew—chew," the desired number of times.

      3. Chew with lips closed Some children cannot voluntarily close lips, which is a sucking reflex. If a child is unable to close lips and chew, place him on his stomach. Then, if he doesn't close his lips, the "precious treat" falls out of his mouth.

      4. Increase the child's diet of chewy foods, hard bread, dry toast, carrots, and potato strips, partially cooked whole green beans, crisp bacon, lamb- and porkchops (bone area with some meat on it), drumsticks, hard cookies, etc.

      5. Gum chewing

         a. Teach gum chewing—use bubble gum. A small piece of gum is given to the child. Before he swallows it, or 30 seconds by the watch, remove the gum. It should be offered daily at the same time. Continue to remove it after 30 seconds for 2 weeks. Then increase the time to 60 seconds for another 2 weeks, making the periods progressively longer thereafter.

         b. Since chewing may not be initially pleasurable, training should not occur at mealtime.

   B. *The Tongue*—the tongue movements are the most involved ones in mastication. Normally, after the food enters the front of of the mouth, the tongue makes a lapping motion—gathering up the food with the tip and carrying it backward quickly under the molar teeth. The food is frequently shifted from one side of the mouth to the other. After it has been lubricated with saliva and masticated, the tongue humps upward and moves backward to thrust the food for swallowing.

1. The food should be placed on top of the tongue, back of the apex.

2. "Paint" syrup or peanut butter inside the upper gum and encourage the child to lick it off.

3. Lateral tongue movements—inside the mouth.
   a. "Paint" the inside of the cheek; first one, then the other with syrup, etc.
   b. Caramels furnish good but difficult practice because of their tendency to get stuck in various parts of the mouth. Smaller caramels can be made by warming and cutting larger pieces into cubes, pressing them around the end of pipe cleaners or paper cylinders as in lollipops, and permitting them to harden with age. This flexible lollipop can be moved easily about the inside of mouth by you.
   c. Bits of cookies placed strategically in the pouch of each cheek.
   d. Place a foreign object—a small piece of adhesive tape—in the cheek of a dry mouth. The tongue, in a defense mechanism, will gravitate toward it.
   e. Apply resistance to the tongue with a wooden tongue depressor or the back of a small plastic spoon. Start off by resisting a movement you know the child can make. For example, if he can hump the back of the tongue, press down *firmly* on it. The child will unconsciously push against it. When training lateral movements, hold the depressor against the side of the tongue and push. After the child develops sufficient strength and you feel his resistance to your movement, reduce the pressure gradually. You will find that instead of pushing against the depressor, the child is following and trying hard to keep up with it. The light pressures, thus, are used as guides to direct the action of the tongue in exercises, the child having learned to keep his tongue against the device.
   f. Brushing—create awareness of the tongue by brushing the tongue with a tongue depressor, a small brush, etc.

Example: if the child is asked to move his tongue to the right and is unable to do so, brush the right side of the tongue briskly. As the area is stimulated, the tongue moves in the direction of the stimulation. Occasionally a child will move the tongue away from the stimulation. If this is consistent, you need only reverse the technique.

4. Projecting the tongue.
   a. Retrieve food on lips—the child should use his tongue, not his hand or sleeve, nor have his lips wiped for him.
   b. Hold lollipop, candy cane, popsicle in front of the mouth (close to lips and gradually moving out) for the tongue tip to touch. Give a good taste before beginning and a small piece as reward when exercises are completed.
   c. At home, the mother can encourage scraping of the bowl and licking the spoon after baking cake, cooking pudding, etc.
   d. Smear upper and/or lower lip with jam to lick.
   e. Fasten a small piece of adhesive tape on a dry lip. See 3.d.
   f. Place cookie bits between lower front teeth and lower lip for child to recover.

5. Drawing tongue in.
   a. Place cookie bits on upper surface of tongue tip.
   b. Resistance—cover the tongue tip with a piece of gauze and pull gently.

6. Lateralizing the tongue—outside the mouth.
   a. Start with 4.a. and gradually move your device toward the corner of the mouth.
   b. Place attractive and good tasting bits of food (candy, sugar, etc.) into the corners of the mouth.

IV. MOVING THE LIPS

A. *Imitation of Movements*

1. Imitation of a hand puppet, an attractive picture of a child, yourself, or himself in the mirror. Introduce such movements as smile, sneer, pucker, disdain, disgust.

B. *Games*—games for opening and closing the mouth.

C. *Movements with Sound*—teach the child to make lip movements combined with sound.

1. The raspberry hum (noisily blowing air through closed lips).

2. Indian War Call (as you say "ah . . . ah . . . ah . . ." the palm of your hand goes back and forth in front of lips).

3. Lip smacking.

4. Kissing.

5. Have the child flip or stroke your lips as you make the "m . . . m . . . m . . ." sound. Then you stroke his lips as he makes the sound.

V.   LEARNING TO KEEP THE MOUTH CLOSED—the pattern of holding the mouth open can become so habutial that the child may have difficulty in remembering to keep it closed. The ability to chew with the lips closed requires separation of jaw and lip functions. (This is also necesary for certain phases of speech.) Lip closure is part of the sucking-swallowing reflex. Some techniques for training:

1. Hold a piece of paper between the lips.

2. Thread a string through a button and place a light weight of some sort, such as a small lead animal, or the other end. Placing the button between the lips and teeth, the child is encouraged to hold the animal up by keeping the lips closed around the button.

3. Thread a rubber band through a button and play a game of "Tug 'o War" in which the child holds the button between the lips and teeth or behind the front teeth while you pull lightly on the rubber band. (This is excellent for strengthening the lips.)

4. Straw sipping.

5. All food should be sucked off the tip of a spoon. To teach this skill, rest the spoon tip on the lower incisors; bring the lips together (with fingers if necessary) over the food.

VI. GAMES TO FURTHER DEVELOP THE ORAL MUSCULATURE

A. *Imitation*

1. Have the children imitate as you perform the various tongue, jaw, and lip movements.

2. Have him imitate you or a hand puppet in a smile, sneer, pucker, show of disdain, or disgust. Or have him imitate pictures that clearly convey these facial and oral expressions.

3. Have him imitate a kitten lapping up food from a saucer. Provide a good tasting fluid in the saucer.

B. *Licking*

1. Have the child lick a popsicle, sucker, or ice cream cone.

C. *Cheek Puffing*

1. Make a game of cheek puffing (the alternate puffing out and pulling in of the cheeks will result in a fore and aft movement of the tongue inside the mouth).

D. *Counting*

1. Use a stop watch, count the number of times per second each child can make the requested movements. (For continuous speech, and adequate speech, the child must be able to raise the tongue many times per second without the assistance of the jaw.)

E. *Variations*—whenever the task permits, have the child perform in a variety of positions, while the child is on the back, stomach, either side, sitting and standing.

1. Developmental order of lingual movements.
   a. Extending tongue out between teeth and lips.
   b. Drawing tongue back into mouth.
   c. Moving tongue to either side.
   d. Raising back of tongue.

Controlled movements are the first prerequisite for speech; however, the child also needs social stimulation. Speech cannot be forced, but as the musculature is developed, suitable conditions for speech should be presented to the child. He must have a sense of belonging in order to arouse in him a desire to communicate; it is the combination of intense auditory stimulation supplying auditory impressions of sufficient magnitude and frequency to "reach" the child and promote a response, adequate speech mechanism, and enriched language experiences that creates speech.

As our non-verbal or slow talkers begin to communicate, they mature through a sequence of articulation patterns which begin at the infantile level. It is well to keep in mind that *speech* does not emerge from silence. Here is the sequence most children follow:

1. Reflex sounds—cry, gulp, sneeze, hiccup, vomit, burp.

2. Whine, whimper, coo.

3. Chuckle, bubble, the raspberry hum.

4. Shriek, laughter.

5. Babble (repetition of syllables, e.g. "abababa"). This stage is auto-stimulating and should be encouraged in the slow-to-speak so that the child retains interest in sound and the vocal practice necessary for later oral skills.

6. Speech—the association of early vocalization, "bye-bye," "ma-ma," "da-da," "ta-ta," with persons, or objects; the development of neologisms—"chu-chu" (train), "wee-wee" (toileting), etc.

During the babbling stage, vowels develop first; some of them, "oo" for instance, are closely associated with the lip movements learned in sucking. Others require only simple gross movement such as opening the mouth for "ah." Consonants follow as the child develops teeth and learns to chew. The very fact that he has teeth requires additional tongue control, or he is apt to bite it. (Chewing adds to the control, as he not only keeps the tongue out of the way of the teeth, but also he uses it to manipulate the food into the proper areas for chewing and swallowing.)

The following activities are suggested to help encourage the child's desire and enhance his ability to communicate:

1. *Phonation*—game of secrets: Tell the child that you are going to say something to him, then make a sound in his ear. Next, the child is asked to say something or just make a noise. This interchange is repeated, and even though he may not understand the language used in explanation, he will comprehend the procedure. If phonation is

weak, loud voluntary sounds will not come suddenly. For a consider-
able time, there may be no response at all. There may be only a glottal
puff which should be rewarded and repeated in the child's ear. Usually
sound production will develop slowly, increase in volume and duration
with repeated practice.

2. *Associate sounds with gross motor movements*—the sounds may be
   vowels, consonants, or a combination of the two. The sound need only
   roughly correspond to the movements. *Examples:*
   a. Rock in a chair—"ah, ah" or humming.
   b. Saw a board—"iiiiiii" or "eeeeeee."
   c. Winding a spool—any vowel on which you rhythmically change
      pitch.
   d. Cranking a toy—"mmmmmmmm."

3. As the child starts to make sounds, imitate his sounds, give him time
   to respond, imitate again. Do not become impatient or pressure the
   child to perform. Give him time—it will come.
   a. If the child shows a real desire to make sounds and tries but cannot
      shape his mouth adequately, some moto-kinesthetic help may be
      needed.*

4. As soon as he will imitate several sounds, pick up his sound, make a
   game of playing the sound back and forth. Then introduce another of
   his familiar sounds to see if he will change from one familiar sound
   to another on cue.

5. Spend weeks playing with the sounds. Elongate them, vary the pitch
   or volume, and then combine: "aaa-eee, aaa-eee."

6. As the child moves into consonant sounds and can imitate several,
   accept less gesture language. Create situations where he must vocalize
   to gain attention or make his desire known. Make a habit of asking,
   "do you want?" one or the other. *Example:* "Do you want milk or
   water?" Then insist on a verbal response—not the whole word, only
   the initial sound or a reasonable facsimile thereof. You can, however, reinforce the correct usage: e.g., if the child says "ba" for
   "ball," reinforce by saying "Yes, it is a ball. Here is the ball."

7. Do not anticipate the child's needs as he shows signs of communicat-
   ing. Watch and wait before stepping in to do the child's "talking" for
   him. Again, accept the initial sound and reinforce.

---

*E. Hill and S. Hawk, *Moto-Kinesthetic Speech Training* (Stanford, Calif.:
Stanford University Press, 1938).

8. Continue the games of imitation, stressing sound combinations and variations in length of sound, pitch, and volume.

9. Accept any verbal efforts and commend the child.

10. Tape recorder games: Have the child listen to brief samples of his own sound production. It is not uncommon for some children to be obsessive about mechanical equipment like the phonograph and tape recorder. Widen and substitute present listening habits so that the obsessional behavior pattern may be lessened and at the same time exploited for teaching purposes.

11. Sing and recite simple repetitious jingles, songs, nursery rhymes to the child. Repeat them over and over. It may seem montonous to you but it is not to the child. He will learn from repetition.

12. Once he is familiar with a few rhymes, encourage him to repeat repetitious words, then later words at the end of a line. *Example:* "Little" in "Ten Little Indians."

13. Teach sounds that animals make. Teach one, give the child plenty of time to become familiar with and sure of it before moving on to the second.

14. Talk to the child. First use words, then short, simple sentences. Time the speech precisely so that he attaches it to the current activity. Verbalize exactly what you are doing if the child is watching, or talk about his movements or what he is doing as he plays or works. *Examples:*
    a. "Down-up"—as child stoops and stands or moves an arm or leg.
    b. "Johnny is moving his arm. He is moving a crayon back and forth, back and forth, back and forth."
    c. "I am cutting paper. These pieces of paper you can paste together to make a picture."

Glossary

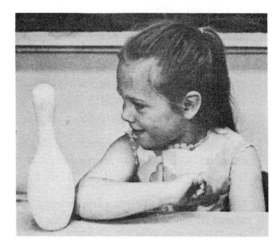

Tasks performed with body parts not normally involved aid the development of body image.

Accommodation: the ocular focusing adjustment for vision at varying distances. It enables us to see objects *clearly* at varying distances.

Auditory: of or relating to hearing.

Bilateral: pertaining to the use of both sides of the body in a simultaneous and parallel fashion.

Binocular: use of both eyes simultaneously.

Body Image: complete awareness of one's own body and its possibilities of movement and performance.

Cephalo-caudal Principle: development begins in the head-neck region and proceeds down through the lower limbs.

Concept: knowledge which at the moment need not be directly perceived through the senses but is the result of the manipulation of previously stored sensory impressions. A concept requires abstraction (the ability to isolate a unit in the whole) and generalization (the ability to recognize that the same "tag" or name may be used for several different objects). *Example:* one might perceive certain properties in a chair, i.e. legs, back, seat, but for a concept one must also become aware of these properties as constituting parts of the general notion of "chairness."

Convergence: the ocular pointing mechanism by which the two eyes are "aimed" at the target. It enables one to see an object singly over varying distances.

Cross-lateral Coordination: the combination or working together of parts on either side of the body in relation to each other.

Cross-lateral Movements: movements requiring the simultaneous use of different limbs on opposite sides of the body, or the moving of the same limbs (as both arms) simultaneously but in opposite directions.

Crossing the Midline: the movement of the eyes, a hand and forearm, or foot and leg across the midsection of the body without involving any other part of the body, i.e. without head turning, trunk twisting or swaying, or without innervation of the opposite limb.

Differentiation: the ability to sort out and use independently different parts of the body in a specific and controlled manner. *Example:* the ability to innervate the muscles of one arm without innervating in a similar fashion the muscles of the other arm or any of the parts of the body not required by the task.

Distractibility: the inability to hold one's attention fixed on a given task for more than a few seconds.

Directionality: the projecting of all directions from the body out into space, right and left, up and down, fore and aft. The child must develop laterality within his own organism and be aware of the right and left sides of his own body before he is ready to or able to project these directional concepts into external space.

Elaboration: embellishment by the addition of variations of associated ideas or movements.

Experimentation: the ability, desire, and willingness of the child to try or test a newly learned movement, or task, or idea to see how many different ways it can be used of itself or in correlation with other movements, tasks, or ideas. Elaboration is the result of experimentation.

Fine Motor Activities: activities or output in which precision in delicate muscle systems is required.

Fixations: the ability of the eyes to point at a given target accurately (ocular marksmanship).

Form Perception: the ability to perceive an arrangement or pattern of elements or parts constituting a unitary whole, wherein the elements are in specific relationships with each other.

Frustration Level: a degree of task difficulty which the child is incapable of performing at a given time.

Generalization: the process of deriving or inducing (a general concept or principle) from particulars. *Example:* the child can categorize objects that are similar and yet different, e.g. recognize many types of chairs as chairs, recognize a square in many settings and media, etc.

Generalized Movement: a wave of movement that sweeps through the whole body. Parts such as arms and legs are moved, not in relationship to their function, but only as an adjunct of the total movement.

Gross Motor Activity: activities or output in which groups of large muscles are used and the factors of rhythm and balance are primary.

Handedness: the choice of hand or side that is to lead in all activities. True handedness grows out of laterality, the inner knowledge of the two sides of one's body and the ability to call forth the one needed for a prescribed task. False handedness is merely a naming of sides, and this is often done by linking one side to a external object such as a ring, memorizing placement of objects in classroom, etc.

Integration: the pulling together and organizing of all of the stimuli which are impinging on the organism at a given moment. It also involves the tying together with the present stimulation, experience variables retained from past activities. The organizing of many individual movements into a complex response.

Kinesthetic: the sense that yields knowledge of the movements of the muscles of the body and position of the joints.

Laterality: complete motor awareness of the two sides of the body.

Midline: the child's own center of gravity. Unless he has a well defined midline as the result of well developed laterality, his space structure will not be stabilized and he may have difficulty orienting himself to his surroundings.

Monocular: the use of one eye while the other eye is shut or covered.

Movement Patterns: the organization of single movements into complex wholes. The movement pattern allows the child to concentrate on the purpose or goal of the movement rather than on how the movement can be made.

Ocular: having to do with the eyes.

Orientation: the child's ability to locate himself in space in relation to the things surrounding him in space and/or in time. Also the ability to stabilize his environment so that it remains more or less constant.

Perception: an experience or sensation combined or integrated with previous experiences which give it added meaning.

Perceptual-Motor: the perceptual-motor process includes input (sensory or perceptual activities) and output (motor or muscular activities). A division of the two is impossible, for anything that happens to one area automatically affects the other. Any total activity includes input, integration, output, and feedback.

Peripheral Vision: visual sensations arising from the visual sense cells lying outside the central (foveal) area of the retina.

Perseveration: the inability to develop a new response to a new or altered stimulus.

Proximo-distal: the direction from the center outward. Movements of large muscle groups lying toward the center of the body develop before the independent movements of parts lying at the extremities. Thus movements of the total arm precede those of the wrist and fingers.

Pursuits: the ability of the eyes to follow a moving target accurately.

Redundancy: the art of presenting the same information to as many of the senses, as simultaneously as possible, in a given task. *Example:* tracing a square on sand paper with the finger. The child *sees* the square, *hears* the movement of this finger across the rough surface, *feels* the tactual contact of his finger with the paper, and also feels the kinesthetic or muscular movements in his hand and arm.

Readiness Skills: those skills, developed by various means, which are necessary for a child to achieve a degree of success in higher levels of learning.

Rigidity: resistance to undertaking a new kind of response.

Space Perception: the direct awareness of the spatial properties of an object, especially in relation to the observer. The perception of position, direction, size, form, distance by any of the senses.

Spatial-temporal Translation: the ability to translate a simultaneous relationship in space into a serial relationship in time, or vice versa. *Example:* the child must recognize the square as a whole when he sees it in space and reproduce it in time as an organized series of lines and angles. To achieve in many of the tasks we set before him, the child must be able to organize his impressions in both of these areas and to shift fluently from one to the other as the situation demands.

Splinter Skill: a restricted approach to a specific problem that exists in isolation, "splintered off" from the remainder of the child's activity. Its usefulness is limited, being adequate for only one type of activity. This isolated response also confuses the child, since he is required to live with two basic learning sets between which there is little or no connection. Also educational skills that have been memorized because they were learned out of context, that is, outside and above the child's performance level. They, too, are isolated facts that the child can neither elaborate nor integrate.

Stimulation Level: the level of activity that demands just enough effort on the child's part to keep him interested and to encourage him to experiment further.

Strabismus: lack of coordination of the eye muscles so that the two eyes do not focus on the same point.

Structuring: the act of arranging an activity in a way that is understandable to the child and conducive to performance, or in other words, arranging the task in such a way that the child will be aware of what is expected of him. Once the task is structured the child should be left on his own to perform without additional cueing.

Tactile or Tactual: having to do with the sense of touch. We use it to express both the child's application of his sense of touch to a given object or task and the use of tactual clues applied to the child by the instructor.

Tactual-kinesthetic: a combination of the sense of touch and the sense of muscle movement.

Time Perception: the awareness of the length of time occupied by a psychological process, of rate of change, of placement in time, of order of occurrence.

Tolerance Level: the level at which the child can perform without any effort and at which he will soon become bored or uninterested.

Unilateral: one sided. The child who is unilateral uses one side of his body and ignores the other.

Variations: minute changes in movement, media, environment, presentation, position, etc.

Visual: pertaining to the use of the eyes.